WITHDRAWN

OPTIMUM NUTRITION
MADE EASY

How to achieve optimum health

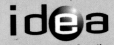

Library Learning Information

To renew this item call:

020 7364 4332

or visit

www.ideastore.co.uk

Created and managed by Tower Hamlets Council

PIATKUS

By The Same Author

'My friend was badly suffering from menopausal sweats/hot flushes – having read *The Optimum Nutrition Bible* I suggested she follow the supplement advice in the book and within 2 weeks she said they'd disappeared! She is still enjoying good health and months later has had no further problems.'

Janette S.

'After reading this book I have been trying to improve my health in the past month by eating better and taking supplements. I was both surprised and pleased to see a rapid reduction in the wrinkly skin under my eyes. My skin is now smooth and "filled out". It has shown me that improving your nutrition can have immediate effects. Thanks Patrick, I've finally woken up to the importance of nutrition.'

N.W.

'I used to have constant pain in my knees and joints, could not play golf or walk more than 10 minutes without resting my legs. Since following your advice my discomfort has decreased 95–100%. It is a different life when you can travel and play golf every day. I never would have believed my pain could be reduced by such a large degree, and no return no matter how much activity in a day or week.'

Ed S.

'In mid-April I had my blood checked and found my cholesterol to be 6.5. I do eat really healthily and felt that my condition was due to hereditary cholesterol rather than dietary factors. A friend had reduced theirs through the supplements recommended in your book, so I thought it was worth a try. Five weeks later I went for a second blood test to find my cholesterol had dropped to 5.1. My GP couldn't believe it! He would not wholeheartedly acknowledge the success, but he didn't knock it either, saying whatever you are taking is working – come back in a year!'

Mike T.

'I feel moved to tell you I consulted you in 1986 with a recurrence of breast cancer. Now, 13 years later, I am pleased to tell you I have just celebrated my seventy-fifth birthday and am fit and well, taking no medication and attending no clinics. I am sure this is in large part due to the advice I received from you.'

Betty L.

'Patrick Holford has given my two girls the mother they deserve instead of the one who had nothing left to give, and my husband back the vibrant person he married and some!!!!! He just now needs to try and keep up with me. My future and that of my daughters and their children will now take a very different path. I wish you every success in spreading the word.'

Dawn V.

Piatkus

First published in Great Britain in 2008 by Piatkus Books

Copyright © Patrick Holford 2008

Reprinted 2008

A CIP catalogue record for this book is available from the British Library

ISBN 978-0-7499-2866-7

Printed and bound in Italy by L.E.G.O. SpA
Designed by MPA Design

Piatkus Books
An imprint of
Little, Brown Book Group
100 Victoria Embankment
London EC4Y 0DY

An Hachette Livre UK Company
www.hachettelivre.co.uk
www.piatkus.co.uk

Picture credits
Photolibrary Group: pp. 10, 19, 35, 44, 46, 68, 88, 95, 98, 121, 124, 136, 142; Alamy: pp. 48, 63, 133, 152; p. 31 Linda Burgess/Redcover.com; p. 111 Tim Evan-Cook/Redcover.com; p. 112 Steve Lupton/Corbis.

Acknowledgements

I am immensely indebted to Susannah Lawson, the highly-talented nutritional therapist and writer, who has helped create this easy to access book from all my material. We would also like to thank the team at Piatkus/Little, Brown who have painstakingly perfected these words to give you a potent and powerful introduction to what is, quite simply, the most important information anyone needs to become and to stay healthy.

Guide to abbreviations, measures and references

Guide to abbreviations and measures

1 gram (g) = 1000 milligrams (mg) = 1,000,000 micrograms (mcg, also written µg).

All vitamins are measured in milligrams or micrograms. Vitamins A, D and E used to be measured in International Units (ius), a measurement designed to standardise the various forms of these vitamins that have different potencies.

6mcg of betacarotene, the vegetable precursor of Vitamin A is, on average, converted into 1mcg of retinol, the animal form of Vitamin A. So, 6mcg of betacarotene is called 1mcgRE (RE stands for retinol equivalent). Throughout this book betacarotene is referred to in mcgRE.

1mcg of retinol (mcgRE) = 3.3ius of Vitamin A
1mcgRE of betacarotene = 6mcg of betacarotene
100ius of Vitamin D = 2.5mcg
100ius of Vitamin E = 67mg
1 pound (lb) = 16 ounces (0z) 2.2lb = 1 kilogram (kg)
1 pint = 0.6 litres 1.76 pints = 1 litre

In this book calories means kilocalories (kcals)

Guide to references and further sources of information

Hundreds of references from respected scientific literature have been used in writing this book. For simplicity, these have not been listed individually but are available in *The New Optimum Nutrition Bible* (also published by Piatkus).

At the end of each chapter or subject, a guide is included for further reading if you want to know more about a particular topic. Scientific studies are also referenced in more detail in these books. You will also find many of the topics touched on in this book covered in detail in my feature articles, available at *www.patrickholford.com*. If you want to stay up to date with all that is new and exciting in this field, I recommend you subscribe to my *100% Health* newsletter, details of which are on the website.

Contents

If you woke up 100% healthy,
how would you know?

I would have *(tick your choices)*:

- ☐ Abundant energy
- ☐ Ideal weight
- ☐ Great skin
- ☐ No pain
- ☐ Happy and motivated mood
- ☐ Sharp mind and memory
- ☐ A strong immune system and be rarely ill
- ☐ Balanced hormones
- ☐ Trouble-free digestion

All this is achievable.

It's putting optimum nutrition into practice.

Find out how you can make all this happen for you...

Introduction

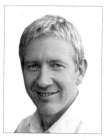

When you buy a car you get a manual, but no such thing occurs for your body. How do you know what to eat to feel great, stay youthful and free from disease? This is the question I've been exploring for the past 30 years, and the reason for setting up the Institute for Optimum Nutrition in 1984. In 1998 I wrote down all we had learnt in the *Optimum Nutrition Bible*, a fully-referenced guide that's sold well over a million copies, and been translated into some twenty languages from Hebrew to Chinese.

The purpose of this book is to make it easy for you to 'cut to the chase' and discover the truth about what to eat to feel great. In this book you will find out exactly what 'optimum nutrition' means, based on three decades of research, tried and tested on hundreds of thousands of people like you. However important you think nutrition is, you will discover that it can literally make the difference between a healthy life and premature death, between feeling just 'all right' and living with more energy than you may have ever experienced, with no risk of the common degenerative diseases from arthritis to cancer.

What you will not find in this book is the usual watered down version of healthy eating guidelines designed not to overly upset the massive and influential multinational food and drug industry. You will not find the basic 'well balanced diet' platitudes that allow most people to think they eat well, yet still suffer from weight gain, low energy, digestive problems, bad skin and other classic signs of sub-optimal nutrition.

For just about every major disease that exists, there's a country that doesn't have it. Why is this? Why, for instance, do us Westerners have a risk for breast or prostate cancer that's more than one hundred times higher than the rural Chinese? It's not genetics – nor is it that we live longer. It's most likely due to simple differences in diet. These are the kind of issues you'll become clear about and, in the process, find out exactly what optimum nutrition really means for you, and what you need to do to achieve it – right down to the food you buy and the supplements to take.

As you read through *Optimum Nutrition Made Easy*, you'll be amazed at how many simple and potent solutions there are to common health problems and, as you apply these principles, you'll be pleasantly surprised at how robust your health and vitality becomes. I've been following these principles for 30 years and can honestly say, at the age of 50, that my energy is as great, my mind probably sharper, my skin better, my weight and health statistics essentially the same as when I was a teenager, and my overall health is definitely better. I cannot remember taking a day off sick – for at least a decade.

This book is for people who want results. It's organised into five parts. In Part One, I explain the basics of optimum nutrition. Part Two is more interactive – there are quizzes to complete for six key aspects of your health to help you determine which particular areas require more focus. Part Three provides some more inspiration for healthy food – plus tips on meeting the changing needs throughout your life, from maximising fertility to feeding babies and children; staying young and beautiful to avoiding the most common degenerative diseases. Then in Part Four, you can put it all together in your own personalised 100% Health Action Plan. And finally, Part Five provides some additional information to help you make optimum nutrition a reality for you.

I wish you the very best of health!

Patrick Holford

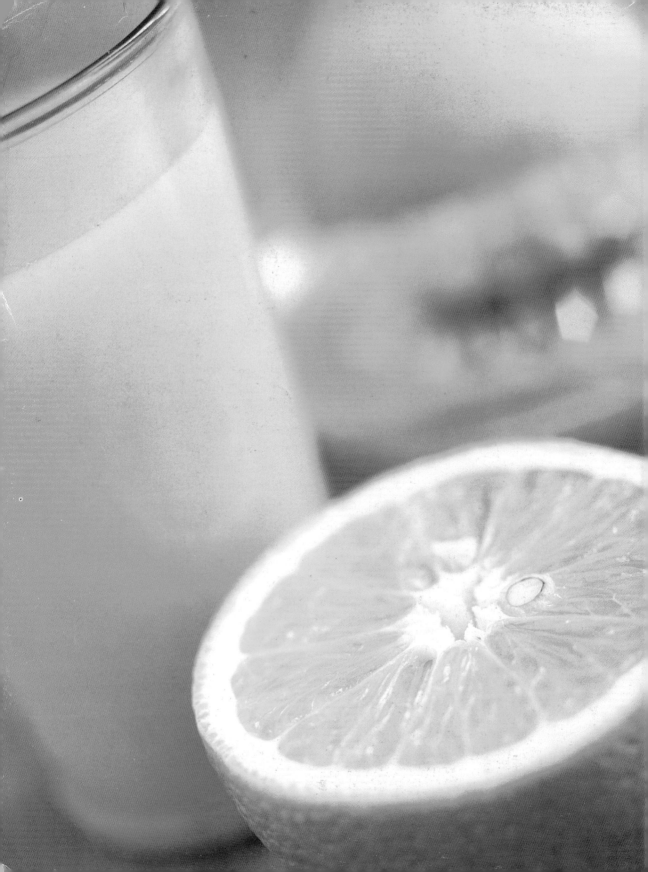

Part One

Getting the Basics Right

1. What Does Optimum Nutrition Mean?

Optimum nutrition is very simply giving yourself the best possible intake of nutrients to allow your body and brain to be as healthy as possible – and to work as well as it can. By nutrients, I mean protein, carbohydrate, essential fats, vitamins, minerals and water – each of which we'll explore in more detail in the coming chapters. These are the substances from which your body is built. For example, your skin renews itself in 21 days, your bones can repair themselves in six weeks and your inner skin, your digestive tract, replaces itself every four days. In five years, you will be an almost completely new person. Your body is an incredible regenerating organism that is constantly self-regulating and rejuvenating. But without the right nutrients, this process becomes impaired. Then you don't replace your body cells quite so accurately – that's called ageing. And with our modern nutrient-lacking diets and endless temptations, maintaining a healthy body is a challenge for everyone.

At the Institute for Optimum Nutrition, we conducted the UK's largest ever survey on diet and health. Some 37,000 people told us what they ate and how they felt. A staggering 85 per cent reported low energy levels, 81 per cent don't have a bowel movement every day, 64 per cent are anxious, 62 per cent are bloated, 56 per cent have dry skin, 45 per cent are depressed, and 64 per cent of women suffer premenstrually. So if you're not feeling in the best of health, you are not alone.

The good news is we know that optimum nutrition can help you to reverse these kind of problems. It can also:

• Improve mental clarity, mood and concentration

• Increase IQ

- Increase physical performance

- Improve quality of sleep

- Improve resistance to infections

- Protect you from disease

- Extend your healthy lifespan

These may sound like bold claims, yet each has been proven by research. And they apply to everyone – irrespective of genetic inheritance.

It's not all in the genes

We are each born with different strengths and weaknesses and different levels of resilience. Some of us have what are popularly called 'good genes' and some of us do not. But does that mean that our health throughout life is predetermined when we are born? The short answer is no!

Let's take breast cancer as an example. Some consider our susceptibility to developing this disease to be determined by our genes. Yet in studies tracking the health of 44,000 sets of twins, 27 per cent of the risk was due to inherited factors. That means that in 73 per cent, the risk is due to external factors such as diet and lifestyle. Alzheimer's is another good example. Only one in 100 cases of this dehabilitating disease is caused by genes. Unless you are the unlucky one per cent, you never need to suffer this fate. This means that your state of health can largely be determined by the way you choose to live.

Even in cases where it's known that someone has a gene that could predispose them to a certain disease, it doesn't mean they will go on to develop that disease. While some genes are set – for example those that determine your eye colour – others can be activated according to the environment in which they find themselves. So if you smoke and drink too much, a disease gene is more likely to be activated. But if you eat well and look after yourself, it may lie dormant for your entire life.

Likewise, if your day-to-day environment is sufficiently hostile (for example, bad diet, pollution, high stress levels) you are more likely to get sick. But if your environment promotes health, then your risk of disease and ill health – no matter what your genetic inheritance – dramatically reduces.

You are unique

There is nobody quite like you. In the same way your genes are unique, your needs are also completely unique and depend on a whole host of factors, from the strengths and weaknesses that you were born with, right up to the effects that your current environment has on you. You only have to look at the tremendous variation in the way we look, and in our talents and personalities, to realise that our nutritional needs are also unlikely to be identical. That's why saying we all need 60mg of Vitamin C each day (which is the UK government's recommended intake for adults) is like saying we all need size ten shoes.

Of course there are many principles that apply to us all as members of the human race – for example, we all need protein, vitamins and minerals; but the actual amount we need varies from individual to individual. Working out your specific needs – your optimum nutrition – and how best to achieve this is what this book will help you establish.

Modern diets are not designed for good health

Before we even start to work out your individual needs, first we must look at your general diet and its contribution – or otherwise – to your health.

As a human being, you are made from approximately two-thirds water, one-quarter protein, and the rest is fat and a few minerals and vitamins. Every single molecule in your body comes from what you eat and drink. Eating the highest quality food in the right quantities helps you to achieve your highest potential for health, vitality and freedom from disease.

Today's diet has drifted a long way from the ideal intake and balance of nutrients. The pie charts opposite show the percentage of calories we consume that come from fat, protein and carbohydrate. While little overall change has occurred throughout 99 per cent of humanity's history, in the last century – particularly the last three decades – we have started eating much more fat, and the wrong kind, much more sugar and refined carbohydrates, more salt and much less fibre. Even the government guidelines fall a long way short of our ancestors' diets or what are generally considered to be ideal dietary guidelines. In fact, they encourage

Ancient and Modern Diets

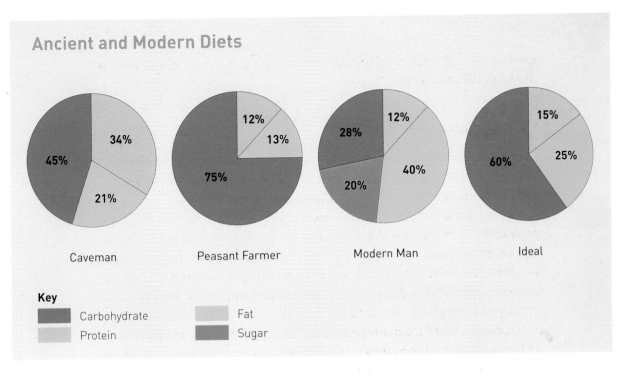

Caveman — 45%, 34%, 21%

Peasant Farmer — 12%, 13%, 75%

Modern Man — 28%, 12%, 40%, 20%

Ideal — 15%, 25%, 60%

Key
- Carbohydrate
- Protein
- Fat
- Sugar

eating more refined, starchy foods – the very foods that promote weight gain, diabetes and heart disease.

Part of the problem is the modern lifestyle. As our lives speed up, we spend less time preparing fresh food and become ever more reliant on processed foods from companies whose main concern is their profit rather than our health. This means food is often refined to last longer, stuffed full of chemicals to look and taste artificially appealing and is stripped of essential nutrients in the process. Society has also become addicted to sugar – today we eat an average 38 kilograms per person per year, compared to just 9 kilograms in 1900. And while the UK government recommends that no more than 10 per cent of calories come from sugar, it does little to discourage us from eating it. Sugar sells, and the more of it we eat, the less room there is for less sweet, low 'GL' carbohydrates (more on this on page 54) that promote energy, weight loss and health.

Since 1984, the Institute for Optimum Nutrition has been researching what a perfect diet would look like. Our conclusions are explained in the next two chapters and summarized on page 43. While for many people, this kind of balance of foods is not going to be achievable overnight, it does give a clear indication of where your diet should be heading.

2. Defining Today's Perfect Diet

Do you want to feel fantastic? Do you want to get the best you can from your diet? Well be prepared to change commonly held views. For example, I'll explain why meat and milk are not ideal dietary staples and actually increase your risk of certain diseases, and why fat doesn't necessarily make you fat, nor increase your risk of heart disease – but sugar does!

Protein: the body's building blocks

The word protein is derived from 'protos', meaning 'first' since protein is the basic material of all living cells. The human body is, for example, approximately 64 per cent water and 22 per cent protein. As well as being vital for growth and the repair of body tissue, protein is used to make hormones, enzymes, antibodies, neurotransmitters and to help transport substances around the body.

While protein forms the building blocks of our body, amino acids are the building blocks of protein. Some 22 different types of amino acids are pieced together in different combinations to make various kinds of protein, in much the same way as letters make words, which combine to make sentences and paragraphs. Of these 22, 16 can by made by your body, but the remaining eight must come from your diet. These eight are therefore termed 'essential' and their balance in the protein of any given food determines its quality, or usability.

The belief that you can only get good-quality protein from animal products is a myth (see Meat and Milk box). Two of the best quality protein foods in terms of amino acid balance are quinoa (a South American grain that you cook like rice, pronounced 'keen-wah') and soya (for example, tofu). And unlike meat, which can contain high levels of saturated fat (for example, 75 per cent of a lamb chop's calories are provided by

Meat and Milk – The Ideal Staples?

The average person in the UK eats over 2lb/900g of meat and drinks four pints of milk a week. The traditional view is that these foods – long-term staples of the British diet – are good for you. But there is growing evidence that the opposite is actually true.

For starters, modern farming methods mean most non-organic meat and milk products contain antibiotics, pesticide residues and high levels of growth hormones. These have all been linked to health risks in humans, including hormone-related cancers and food poisoning from antibiotic-resistant superbugs.

Meat and dairy consumers also have a low health rating. The risk of heart disease and cancer – particularly cancer of the stomach and colon – is directly related to meat consumption, as are other digestive diseases such as diverticulitis, colitis and appendicitis. According to research from Surrey University, a meat-eater is likely to visit the doctor, or be admitted to hospital, twice as often as a vegetarian, and is likely to start suffering from degenerative diseases ten years earlier.

A high consumption of milk and dairy products is even more likely to result in cardiovascular disease. Milk consumption is also strongly linked with increased risk for breast and prostate cancers (see page 127). And in babies, early exposure increases the likelihood of developing allergies – it's even been linked with increased risk of infant-onset diabetes.

But what may really surprise you is that drinking too much milk – as well as eating too much meat – may increase your risk of osteoporosis. This is because despite its calcium content, the protein milk contains makes the body more acidic. And when the body becomes acidic, it uses alkaline bone minerals such as calcium as a buffer. One 12-year study found that women who drank two or more glasses of milk a day actually had a 45 per cent higher risk of hip fractures and a 5 per cent higher risk of forearm fractures than women who drank less. The good news is that seeds, nuts and green vegetables like kale and broccoli provide more calcium and also other beneficial minerals lacking in milk, such as magnesium, chromium, manganese and selenium.

From the current evidence, neither meat nor milk should be staple foods if you really want to pursue optimum nutrition. But this is no loss – not only is it possible to have a healthy diet without including dairy produce and meat, it's also almost certainly going to decrease your risk of the common killer diseases. For meat-lovers who really don't want to go vegetarian, eat meat no more than three times a week (but choose only organic and lean meats and free-range chicken), and substitute fish and vegetarian protein foods such as beans, lentils and quinoa. For milk, substitute soya, oat or rice milk, often enriched with calcium, or buy organic milk. If you suspect you might be allergic, stay off all dairy produce for 14 days. If it makes no difference, limit your intake of milk to two pints a week.

saturated fat), vegetable sources tend to contain more beneficial fats, plus other nutrients which make them less acid forming and better for you than meat.

It is therefore best to limit meat to three meals a week. Other good protein sources include fish, free-range eggs, grains and pulses, which means beans, lentils, nuts and seeds. Many vegetables – especially 'seed' foods such as runner beans, peas, corn or broccoli – contain both protein and lots of anti-ageing antioxidants.

Overall, protein – lean meat, fish, eggs and pulses – should make up about one-sixth to a quarter of what you eat, or around 15 to 25 per cent of your total calorie intake. (The higher percentage helps promote weight loss.) You can achieve this by following the guidelines below.

Protein: optimum nutrition guidelines

• Eat two servings of beans, lentils, quinoa, tofu (soya), 'seed' vegetables or other vegetable protein, or one small serving of meat, fish or cheese, or a free-range egg, every day.

• Reduce your intake of dairy products and avoid them altogether if you are allergic, substituting soya, oat or rice milk.

• Reduce other sources of animal protein, choosing lean meat or wild or organic fish and eating no more than three servings a week of meat, and three of fish.

• Eat organic whenever possible, to minimise your exposure to toxic and hormone-disrupting chemicals.

Carbohydrate: fuel for energy

Carbohydrate is your main fuel source – it provides energy for you to go about your life and energy for your body to carry on all its incredible work behind the scenes. This vital energy source comes in two forms: 'fast releasing', as in sugar, honey, malt, sweets and most refined foods; and 'slow releasing', as in whole grains, vegetables and most fresh fruits.

Slow-releasing carbohydrates are often called 'complex carbohydrates' because their structure is nutritionally complex and includes fibre – this helps to slow down the release of energy in these foods. By contrast, fast-

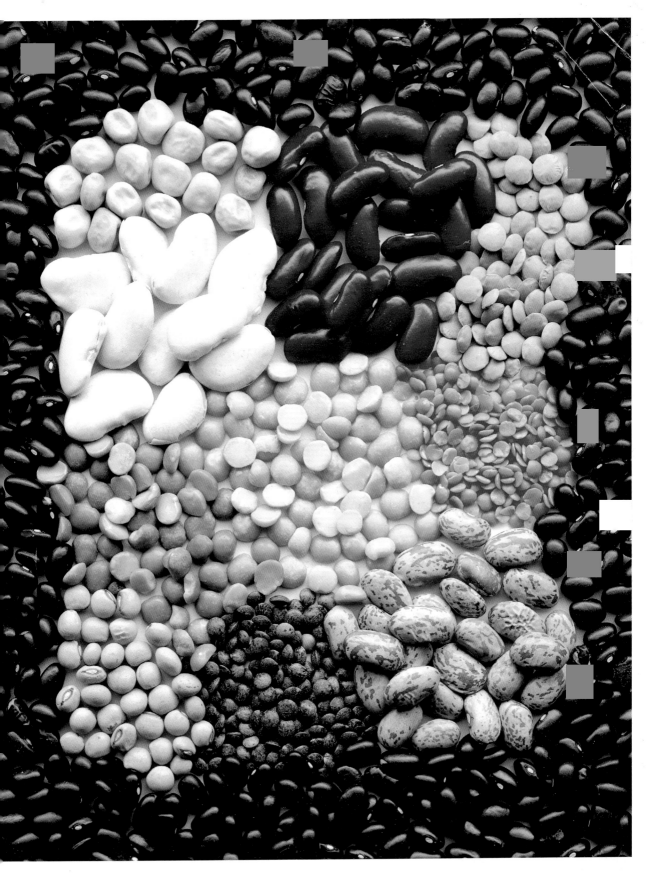

releasing carbohydrates contain simple types of sugar which need little digestion – for example refined white bread or white rice, where the fibre and many of the nutrients have been removed in processing.

Whatever the type of carbohydrate, it's all digested down into its basic energy units – primarily glucose, which is direct fuel for your body cells. Fast-releasing foods release their glucose quicker, giving you a sudden burst of energy. The downside is that after the high comes a slump – that's why you can feel tired or hungry again and crave sweet foods not long after eating a piece of cake or a biscuit. Slow-releasing carbohydrates, on the other hand, do what their name suggests – release their glucose slower, so you get a sustained flow of energy over a longer period. We call these low 'Glycemic Load' (or low GL) foods because they keep your blood sugar level, and your energy more even.

By now you should be getting the idea that slow-releasing carbohydrates are a better option if you want to maintain stable energy levels. Fast-releasing carbohydrates also tend to be refined, for example foods made with sugar and white flour, and they lack the vitamins and minerals needed for the body to properly digest and make use of the fuel they provide. This is why relying mostly on fast-releasing carbohydrates for energy can give rise to health problems such as fatigue, weight gain and even diabetes.

What this means in terms of food choices is that wholegrains are better for you than refined grains – so instead of 'white' carbohydrates, choose brown rice, wholegrain wheat, granary or rye bread, wholemeal pasta, oat cereals and oat cakes. As explained in the protein section earlier, beans, lentils and grains such as quinoa contain protein as well as complex carbohydrates, so they are excellent sources of slow-releasing energy, making you feel fuller for longer. And fresh fruit and vegetables are also a good fibre- and nutrient-rich source of low GL carbohydrates.

Fruit contains a type of sugar called 'fructose', which takes longer for the body to break down than foods made with refined white sugar. This is why fruit makes a more nutritious and energising snack than sugary foods. However, some fruit – like bananas and raisins – contain faster-releasing sugars and are best kept to a minimum if your energy tends to yoyo, or if you want to lose weight. Likewise, fruit juice isolates the sweet part and discards the fibre in the fruit, so it's converted more quickly to energy in the body. It's therefore better to eat your fruit rather than drink it, but if you do, dilute 50/50 with water to slow down its absorption.

Overall, slow-releasing carbohydrate foods – fresh fruit, vegetables, pulses and whole grains – should make up half to two-thirds of what you eat, or around 50 to 65 per cent of your total calorie intake. You can achieve this by following the guidelines below.

Carbohydrate: optimum nutrition guidelines

- Eat whole foods – whole grains, lentils, beans, nuts, seeds, fresh fruit and vegetables – and avoid refined, white and overcooked foods.

- Eat four or five servings of vegetables a day, including dark green, leafy and root vegetables such as watercress, carrots, sweet potatoes, broccoli, Brussels sprouts, spinach, green beans or peppers, either raw or lightly cooked.

- Eat three or more servings a day of fresh fruit, preferably apples, pears, oranges, plums and/or berries.

- Eat four or more servings a day of whole grains such as rice, rye, oat flakes and oat cakes, corn and quinoa as cereal, breads, pasta or pulses.

- Avoid any form of sugar, added sugar, and white or refined foods.

- Dilute fruit juices and only eat dried fruit infrequently in small quantities.

The fats of life

Fat phobics beware. Avoiding all fat is actually bad for your health. The essential types of fat reduce risk of cancer, heart disease, allergies, Alzheimer's disease, arthritis, eczema, depression, fatigue, PMS – the list of symptoms and diseases associated with deficiency is growing every year.

The human brain is 60 per cent fat and one-third of this should come from essential fats if you want to achieve your full potential for health and happiness. But unless you go out of your way to eat the right kinds of fat-rich foods, such as seeds, nuts and oily fish, the chances are that you are not getting enough good fat. Most people in the Western world eat too much saturated fat – found mostly in meat, dairy and processed foods – promoting weight gain.

- Flax seeds
- Hemp seeds
- Walnuts
- Pumpkin seeds
- Sunflower seeds
- Soya beans
- Sesame seeds
- Almonds
- Anchovies
- Sardines
- Pilchards
- Wild salmon
- Mackerel
- Free-range Omega-3 eggs

- Fresh cold-pressed vegetable oils (e.g. olive)

- Coconut oil/butter
- Butter
- Eggs

- Milk
- Cheese
- Roasted nuts and seeds
- Refined oils

- Deep fried foods
- Browned or burnt foods
- Hydrogenated fats

Fats that Kill

Fats essential to health

The reason that fresh nuts, seeds and oily fish are good for you is because, along with other vital nutrients, they contain beneficial 'polyunsaturated' fats called Omega 3 and Omega 6. Common signs of deficiency in these essential fats are dry skin, dandruff or flaky scalp, poor memory, PMS and depression.

Both Omega 3 and 6 fats can be found in flax, hemp and pumpkin seeds. When you eat these, the body converts the fats they contain into their more active forms – for Omega 3, these are called EPA, DPA and DHA; for Omega 6, it's GLA. You can also find these active forms in certain foods. Oily fish such as anchovies, salmon, sardines and mackerel contain the active Omega 3 fats EPA, DPA and DHA. These are a better source than relying on flax seeds or pumpkin seeds. This is because only about 5 per cent of what's in flax seeds is converted into EPA, and even less into DHA, which is literally what your brain is built from. So it's best to both eat oily fish, flax and pumpkin seeds and to supplement Omega 3-rich fish oils. Oils of evening primrose and borage contain the active Omega 6 fat GLA. (See chart opposite.)

Most of us need daily sources of both the original essential fats and their more active forms. Eating fresh nuts and seeds plus oily fish will provide a good balance. If deficiency symptoms such as dry skin or hormonal issues continue to be an issue, add in some extra plant oils such as borage via a daily supplement.

Omega 3		Omega 6	
• Flax (linseed)	EPA, DPA & DHA	• Corn	GLA
• Hemp	• Salmon	• Safflower	• Evening primrose oil
• Pumpkin	• Mackerel	• Sunflower	• Borage (starflower) oil
• Walnut	• Herring	• Sesame	• Blackcurrant seed oil
	• Sardines		
	• Anchovies		
	• Marine algae		
	• Eggs		

The best fats for cooking

Polyunsaturated oils such as seed oils or even sunflower oils are not a good choice for cooking because they are easily damaged when heated, creating harmful molecules called oxidants. The best type of oil to cook with is the more stable monounsaturated variety – of which olive oil is the best source.

Coconut oil is an even better option because despite being a saturated fat, its chemical structure is slightly different to other saturated cooking fats such as butter or lard (meat fat), and the body is therefore better able to utilise it – for energy, rather than turning it into body fat.

Avoid harmful fats

As we've established, eating a lot of meat or dairy produce provides too much saturated fats, so red meat and hard cheese are best limited to no more than three to four portions a week (see page 18 for healthier protein sources).

Processed or refined vegetables oils can also be bad for you because this can change the nature of the oil. For example, when making margarine, vegetable oils go through a process called hydrogenation to make them hard so you can spread rather than pour them. Hydrogenated fats confuse the body and block the uptake of other healthy polyunsaturated fats, so they are best avoided. Sources include some margarines and many processed foods, so check ingredients lists on labels carefully.

Frying is another way to damage otherwise healthy oils. This then damages your body when you eat fried, browned or burnt foods – so these are best kept to a minimum. Instead of frying, steam-fry foods. (Turn to page 106 for healthier ways to cook.)

The Benefits of Olive Oil

While olive oil contains no appreciable amounts of the essential Omega 3 and only a little Omega 6 fat, much of it is cold-pressed and unrefined. This makes it better for you than refined vegetable oils like the sunflower oil you can buy in the supermarket. Also, while there is a strong association between a high intake of saturated fats – mainly from meat and dairy products – and cardiovascular disease, the reverse is true for olive oil. People in Mediterranean countries, whose diets include large quantities of olive oil, have a lower risk of cardiovascular disease.

Overall, fat – mostly the essential variety from oily fish, nuts and seeds – should make up about one-fifth to a quarter, or around 20 to 25 per cent, of your total calorie intake. Since there's twice as many calories in a gram of fat than a gram of protein or carbohydrate, this will look like one- eighth of what you eat. You can achieve this by following the guidelines below.

Fat: optimum nutrition guidelines

• Eat seeds and nuts – the best seeds are flax, hemp, pumpkin, sunflower and sesame. You get more goodness out of them by grinding them first and sprinkling them on cereal, soups and salads.

• Eat oily fish – a serving of anchovies, sardines, mackerel or salmon two or three times a week provides a good source of Omega 3 fats.

• Use seed oils – choose a cold-pressed oil blend for salad dressings and other cold uses, such as drizzling on vegetables instead of butter.

• Minimise your intake of fried food, processed food and saturated fat from meat and dairy produce.

Fruit and vegetables: five-star health benefits

Every time you eat a vegetable or piece of fruit, you are receiving a vast cocktail of anti-ageing nutrients that will influence your health for the better. As well as complex carbohydrates, fibre, vitamins and minerals, natural foods also contain substances called phytochemicals (phyto means plant in Greek). These help to promote health and prevent disease – which is why the UK government encourages us all to have at least 'five a day'. I recommend seven a day, for example fruit with breakfast and two fruit snacks, and two servings of veg, making up half of what's on your plate, with each main meal.

So far, more than a hundred different phytochemicals have been identified and more are being discovered all the time. Some you may be familiar with – for example lycopene in tomatoes helps to prevent cancer – but there are many others which also act to protect your body from the damage of day-to-day life, support a healthy immune system or help to stabilise hormones. Here are some examples:

Allium compounds – these are found in garlic, onions, leeks, chives and shallots and have been found to have protective effects against cancer and heart disease, and also to help lower cholesterol and homocysteine (more on this on page 123) and thin the blood.

Anthocyanidins and proanthocyanidins – these are particularly rich in berries, cherries and grapes and are reputedly healing for gout and certain types of arthritis.

Bioflavonoids – as well as being potent antioxidants, these substances enhance the beneficial actions of Vitamin C, can be antibacterial and strengthen blood vessels (e.g. to help prevent varicose veins or bleeding gums). The best food sources are citrus fruit, berries, broccoli, cherries, grapes, papaya, cantaloupe melon, plums and tomatoes. Red grapes are also rich in resveratrol, one of the most potent antioxidants, concentrated in red wine.

Carotenoids – as the name implies, carotenoids are rich in carrots, but they are also rich in other fruit and vegetables including sweet potato, watercress and peas. They help to slow down the ageing process.

Chlorophyll – this is the substance that makes green plants green. Chlorophyll-rich foods like wheat grass, seaweeds and green vegetables help to 'build' the blood and have been shown to help protect against cancer, radiation, germs and help heal wounds.

Curcumin – this is especially high in turmeric, the yellow spice in curry powder, which is a potent antioxidant and pain-killer.

Ellagic acid – present in strawberries, grapes and raspberries, ellagic acid neutralises cancer-causing toxins before they can damage cells.

Glucosinolates – these are one of the most important anti-cancer and liver-friendly nutrients found in food. Evidence suggests food sources – such as tenderstem broccoli and Brussels sprouts – can reduce risk for lung cancer, stomach cancer, colo-rectal cancer and probably breast cancer.

Lutein – this is a powerful antioxidant found in many fruit and vegetables and is particularly beneficial for maintaining healthy eyesight. The best sources are green leafy vegetables such as cabbage, spinach, broccoli, cauliflower and kale.

Quercitin – this powerful anti-inflammatory agent is particularly rich in red onions and berries, especially cranberries and strawberries, as well

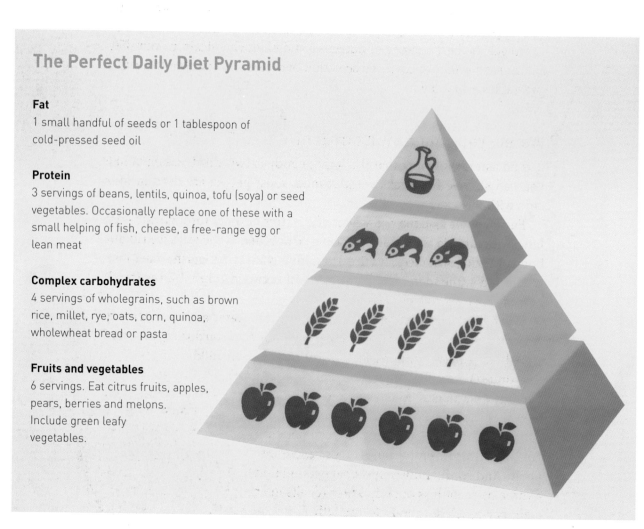

The Perfect Daily Diet Pyramid

Fat
1 small handful of seeds or 1 tablespoon of cold-pressed seed oil

Protein
3 servings of beans, lentils, quinoa, tofu (soya) or seed vegetables. Occasionally replace one of these with a small helping of fish, cheese, a free-range egg or lean meat

Complex carbohydrates
4 servings of wholegrains, such as brown rice, millet, rye, oats, corn, quinoa, wholewheat bread or pasta

Fruits and vegetables
6 servings. Eat citrus fruits, apples, pears, berries and melons. Include green leafy vegetables.

as apples – and can be very effective at easing the symptoms of hayfever, eczema and asthma as well as improving the health of blood vessels and connective tissues. Onions and garlic also help to boost the body's glutathione levels, a potent anti-ageing antioxidant.

These are just a fraction of the phytochemicals in fruits and vegetables. As you may have noticed, the different compounds are commonly related to different colours – anti-ageing carotenoids predominantly in orange and yellow foods, blood-building chlorophyll in green leafy vegetables, anti-inflammatory quercetin in blue and red berries and cancer-killing glucosinolates in crunchy green vegetables. Bright yellow spices such as turmeric and mustard are also excellent natural anti-inflammatories, reducing pain and swelling.

To get the best balance of nutrients and phytochemicals in your diet, aim to eat a rainbow-coloured selection of at least six different fruits and vegetables every day.

Water: your most vital nutrient

It is an astonishing fact that the human body is two-thirds water. While you can survive for weeks without food, most people are dead in four days without water.

Each day, we lose the equivalent of 1.5 litres of water through our skin, lungs, gut and via the kidneys as urine. This is one of the ways we rid our body of toxic substances. It's therefore important to replenish what's lost, with a recommended daily fluid intake of between 1.5 to 2 litres (that's equivalent to six to eight glasses).

As well as transporting toxins for excretion, water acts as a delivery system, a lubricant and a temperature regulator, so if you don't get enough your body simply cannot function optimally. Even mild dehydration can lead to constipation, headaches, lethargy and mental confusion, and increases the risk of urinary tract infections. When just one per cent of body fluids is lost, body temperature goes up and concentration becomes more difficult. And sports nutritionists have found that a three per cent loss of body water results in an eight per cent loss in muscle strength.

FIND OUT MORE
Read *Patrick Holford's New Optimum Nutrition Bible* and *The Optimum Nutrition Cookbook* (published by Piatkus).

Seven Easy Ways to Boost Your Water Intake

Water can be an acquired taste, so you may find it hard to go from drinking none to drinking 2 litres in the space of a few days. Like getting into any good habit, it makes sense to start incorporating small measures first then build up slowly to your goal.

- Put a glass of water by your bed and drink it when you wake up.

- Carry a 500ml bottle of water around to sip throughout the day (when you get used to this, you can refill half-way through the day and boost your intake to 1 litre).

- Dilute fruit juices 50/50 with water.

- Make water more exciting by flavouring it with fresh lemon, lime, ginger, mint or have it hot as a herb or fruit tea.

- Fruit and vegetables consist of around 90 per cent water. Two pieces of fruit and two servings of vegetables can provide 500ml of water (double that and you get a litre!).

- When you feel hungry, drink a glass of water – thirst is often mistaken for hunger.

- Always have a glass of water with a coffee and two glasses of water with every alcoholic drink.

Drinking fluids throughout the day is therefore essential to good health. Ideally, this should be pure, filtered water or natural mineral water (see page 38) or herbal teas. But juices and squashes still count. And even caffeinated drinks like tea, coffee and colas – although not recommended – can contribute towards your daily fluid intake. For every mug or glass you consume, two-thirds can be used by your body as water.

While drinking plenty of water is good for your health, beware of drinking too much. Much more than 2 litres a day can actually tax the kidneys and lead to over-hydration, unless you are exercising heavily.

3. Vitamins and Minerals: From A to Zinc

Vitamins and minerals are needed in much smaller amounts than fat, protein or carbohydrate, but they are no less important. These 'micro-nutrients' control billions of vital actions in your body every single second of your life. They do this by activating substances called 'enzymes' which orchestrate all your body processes. For example, as soon as you eat something, enzymes start working to break the food down so you can digest it, then different kinds of enzymes will take over to utilise the nutrients in the food to turn them into energy, repair your skin, make your hair grow, and so on. Every single vitamin and mineral is needed to make this happen – otherwise the food would just sit in your stomach and do nothing.

These essential nutrients are involved in every function of your body. If you are deficient, your body will not work as efficiently as it could.

Vital vitamins

Vitamins are needed to balance hormones, produce energy, boost the immune system, make healthy skin and protect the arteries; they are vital for the brain, nervous system and every single body process. Vitamins A, C and E are antioxidants: they slow down the ageing process and protect the body from cancer, heart disease and pollution. B and C vitamins are vital for turning food into mental and physical energy. Vitamin D, found in milk, eggs, fish and meat, helps control calcium balance for healthy bones, and promotes healthy immunity, protecting you from cancer and colds. It can also be made in the skin in the presence of sunshine. B and C vitamins are richest in fresh fruit and vegetables. Vitamin A comes in two forms: retinol, the animal form found in meat, fish, eggs and dairy produce; and betacarotene, found in yellow and orange fruit and vegetables. Vitamin E is found in seeds, nuts and their oils, and helps protect essential fats from going rancid.

Miraculous minerals

Like vitamins, minerals are essential for just about every body function. Calcium, magnesium and phosphorus help make up the bones and teeth. Nerve signals, vital for the brain and muscles, depend on calcium, magnesium, sodium and potassium. Oxygen is carried in the blood to every cell by an iron compound. Chromium helps control blood sugar levels. Zinc is essential for all body repair, renewal and development. Selenium and zinc help boost the immune system. Brain function depends on adequate magnesium, manganese, zinc and other essential minerals. These are but a few of thousands of key roles that minerals play in human health.

We need large daily amounts of calcium and magnesium, which are found in vegetables such as kale, cabbage and root vegetables. They are also abundant in nuts and seeds. Calcium alone is found in large quantities in dairy produce. Fruit and vegetables provide lots of potassium and small amounts of sodium, which is the right balance. All 'seed' foods – which include seeds, nuts, lentils and dried beans, as well as peas, broad beans, runner beans, and whole grains – are good sources of iron, zinc, manganese and chromium. Selenium is abundant in nuts, seafood, seaweed and seeds.

More on individual vitamins and minerals – what they do in the body and the best food sources – can be found in the Nutrient Fact Files on page 154.

Team players

As we're starting to see, vitamins and minerals don't work in isolation – they work together in teams (or in synergy) to help your body function. Some nutrients simply will not work on their own. Vitamin B6, for example, is useless in the body until it is converted into its active form, which is a job done by an enzyme that requires zinc and magnesium. If you are zinc or magnesium deficient and take a Vitamin B6 supplement to help relieve premenstrual syndrome (PMS), it will not make any difference. Studies have shown that giving women zinc, magnesium and B6 together relieves the symptoms of PMS much more effectively.

continued on page 34

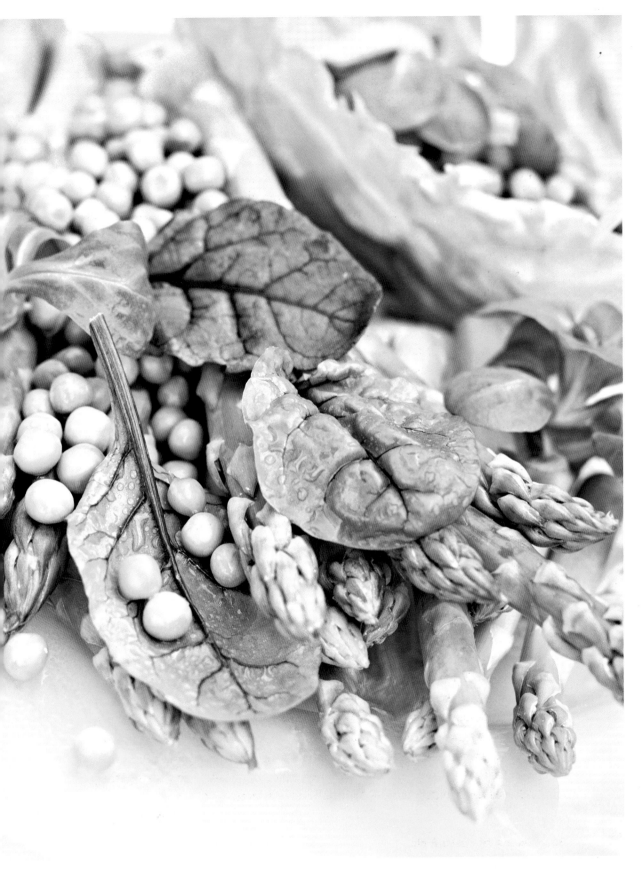

Why Supplements are Necessary

Every survey of eating habits conducted in Britain since the 1980s shows that even those who said they ate a balanced diet fail to eat anything like the European, American or World Health Organisation Recommended Daily Allowances (RDAs). What is more, the RDAs of vitamins and minerals are set by governments to prevent deficiency diseases such as scurvy or rickets, rather than to ensure optimal health. And there is a big difference between a lack of illness and the presence of wellness.

Why, you may wonder, does a good diet not contain all the vitamins and minerals we need for health. Studies show us that nutrient levels in food are falling – there are less vitamins and particularly minerals in fresh produce today, for example, than in the eighties. This is partly due to intensive farming on nutrient-depleted soils and also storing 'fresh' food for longer (for instance, oranges may take four to five months from picking to appearing on your supermarket shelf). Refining food (i.e. turning brown into white) also strips away valuable nutrients. In wheat, for example, 25 nutrients are removed in the refining process that turns it into white flour, yet only five (iron, B1, B2, B3 and folic acid) are replaced. On average, 87 per cent of the essential minerals zinc, chromium and manganese are also lost. We just don't eat what our ancestors ate.

The result of a sub-optimum intake of nutrients is a sub-optimum state of health. Most people put up with feeling 'all right' – accepting the odd cold, headache or mouth ulcer and having low energy, poor digestion, depression and so on as normal.

Yet there are hundreds of scientific studies published in respected medical journals which prove that increasing intake of vitamins and minerals above RDA levels can boost immunity, enhance IQ, reduce birth defects, improve childhood development, reduce colds, stop PMS, improve bone density, balance moods, reduce aggression, increase energy, reduce the risk of diabetes, cancer and heart disease and promote a long and healthy life. If you'd like to see the evidence, go to *www.patrickholford.com* and click on supplements.

Back in 1982 at the Institute for Optimum Nutrition, we did our own study where we put 76 volunteers on a six-month supplement programme. At the end of this time, 79 per cent reported a definite improvement in energy, 60 per cent spoke of better memory and mental alertness, 66 per cent felt more emotionally balanced, 57 per cent had fewer colds and infections and 55 per cent had better skin.

The evidence is clear that you can improve your health in many areas by increasing your intake of vitamins and minerals. That's why I recommend you ensure your diet is as nutrient rich as it possibly can be. But we also know that even a good diet will not give the optimum amount of nutrients, which is why I recommend that you take supplements (see Chapter 5).

Nutrients	RDA	Average Diet	Good Diet	Shortfall	ODA
Vitamin A (mcg)	800	900	1500	shortfall 1000	2500
Vitamin D (mcg)	5	3.5	†15	shortfall 15	30
Vitamin E (mg)	10	14	50	shortfall 200	250
Vitamin C (mg)	60	100	200	shortfall 1800	2000
Vitamin B1 (mg)	1.4	2	5	shortfall 30	35
Vitamin B2 (mg)	1.6	2.18	5	shortfall 30	35
Vitamin B3 (mg)	18	39.6	50	shortfall 50	100
Vitamin B5 (mg)	6	2.175	20	shortfall 80	100
Vitamin B6 (mg)	2	3.1	5	shortfall 20	25
Folic Acid (mcg)	200	325.5	400	shortfall 200	600
Vitamin B12 (mcg)	1	5.95	10	shortfall 15	25
Biotin (mcg)	150	36.5	100	shortfall 50	150
GLA* (Ω6) (mg)	-	20	50	shortfall 50	100
EPA/DPA/DHA* (Ω3) (mg)	-	60	400	shortfall 600	1000
Calcium (mg)	800	(800:Good Diet)	912.5	shortfall 200	1000
Iron (mg)	14	12.8	15	shortfall 5	20
Magnesium (mg)	300	272	350	shortfall 150	500
Zinc (mg)	15	9.3	10	shortfall 10	20
Iodine (mcg)	150	193.5	240	shortfall 60	300
Selenium* (mcg)	-	40	50	shortfall 50	100
Chromium* (mcg)	-	50	70	shortfall 30	100
Manganese* (mcg)	-	3	6	shortfall 4	10

Key

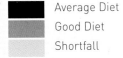

Average Diet

Good Diet

Shortfall

RDA = Recommended Daily Allowance

ODA = Optimum Daily Allowance (diet plus supplements)

* Items marked with an asterisk have no RDA

† Includes Vitamin D created by 20 minutes sun exposure per day.
More Vitamin D may be needed in winter.

How Diets Compare This chart shows the levels of vitamins, minerals and essential fats the average diet – and a good diet – can provide. You can also see how they deliver in terms of the 'RDA' (the government's recommended daily allowance) – and how both fall short of the 'ODA' (optimum daily allowance) that's needed for optimum health. The shortfall is worth supplementing.

The vast majority of research in nutrition, however, has looked at the effects on health of a single nutrient. The results are not comparable with the effects of giving a person optimum nutrition, or the right balance of all essential nutrients. For instance, there is little evidence that individual vitamins or minerals can increase IQ scores in children. However, giving a combination of all vitamins and minerals has consistently been shown to produce a four- to seven-point increase in children's IQ scores.

Antioxidants: disarming the bad guys

Antioxidants are nutrients that help to protect your body from damage. While drinking too much booze, smoking and eating a bad diet harm your body, damage is also caused by everyday essential activities such as breathing, digesting food or fighting infections. This is because oxygen – involved in every body process in every cell, every second of every day – is chemically reactive. It becomes easily unstable and capable of 'oxidising' neighbouring molecules, which can damage cells and trigger ageing, inflammation and even diseases such as cancer.

Unstable oxygen molecules – called 'oxidants' or 'free radicals' – are also present in pollutants (e.g. from industrial processes, cigarette smoke or exhaust fumes) and in fried, burnt and/or barbecued foods.

The good news is the body has an inbuilt repair system, but this needs particular nutrients to power the antioxidant enzymes that disarm the oxidants. The main players are Vitamins A, C, E and betacarotene, the precursor of Vitamin A that is found in fruit and vegetables, plus the minerals zinc and selenium. But you also need the antioxidant nutrients called coenzyme Q10, alpha-lipoic acid, glutathione and resveratrol, the secret ingredient in red wine, for maximum antioxidant protection.

The balance between your intake of antioxidants and your exposure to oxidants may literally be the balance between life and death. You can tip the scales in your favour by making simple changes to your diet and by supplementing antioxidant nutrients (see page 85 for more on this).

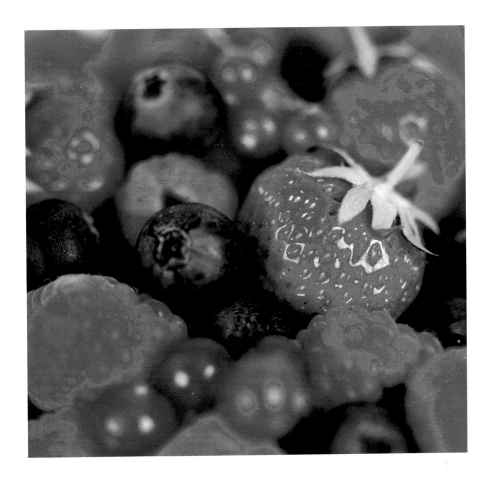

Summary

Vitamins and minerals are essential for every function in the body and also for protecting us from ageing and disease. Research has found that even those eating good diets fail to get all the nutrients needed for basic good health, let alone optimum health. And the food we buy today has lower levels of nutrients than in previous decades, due in part to intensive farming and the trend for eating refined foods. Ensuring your diet is nutrient rich is therefore essential, as is taking a multinutrient supplement to make up the shortfall. Refer to Chapter 5 for diet tips to boost your vitamin and mineral intake, and also what and how to supplement for extra essential nutrients.

FIND OUT MORE
Read *Patrick Holford's New Optimum Nutrition Bible* (published by Piatkus).

4. Anti-nutrients – What to Avoid

Optimum nutrition is not just about what you eat – what you avoid is equally important. Since the 1950s, more than 3,500 man-made chemicals have found their way into our food, along with pesticides, antibiotics and hormone residues. As well as being toxic, many of these chemicals are also 'anti-nutrients', in that they stop beneficial nutrients being absorbed and used by our bodies.

Many of today's diseases are caused just as much by an excess of anti-nutrients as by a deficiency of beneficial nutrients. Take cancer, for example. Three-quarters of all cancers are associated with over-exposure to anti-nutrients, be it from pesticides and other hormone-disrupting chemicals, cigarettes or pollution.

Each year in the UK alone we now get through a staggering quarter of a million tons of food chemicals, 6 billion alcoholic drinks, 75 billion cigarettes, 80 million prescriptions for painkillers and 50 million prescriptions for antibiotics. In addition, 50,000 chemicals are released into the environment by industry and 400 million litres of pesticides and herbicides are sprayed onto food and pastures.

These anti-nutrients also increase our need for beneficial nutrients. If you drink or smoke, you need more Vitamin C to maintain the same levels as someone who doesn't, for example. If you live in a city, exposure to pollution increases your need further.

The first stage in reducing your anti-nutrient load is identifying the key offenders. Then you can take steps to reduce your exposure – and where that is not possible, boost levels of beneficial nutrients that can offer you some protection.

The pesticide problem

Labelling on food does not tell you everything. Unless you eat only organic food, one in three of all the foods you buy contains traces of pesticides. In fact, the amount of fruit and vegetables consumed by the average person in a year has the equivalent of up to 4.5 litres, or one gallon, of pesticides sprayed on it.

Many pesticides are known to be cancer causing, linked to birth defects or decreased fertility, and toxic to the brain and nervous system. Pesticide exposure is also associated with depression, memory decline, aggressive outbursts and Parkinson's disease.

You may be wondering why the government allows pesticides in foods, if they are so harmful. The argument given is that at very low levels they are not harmful to humans, yet the tests used to establish the safety levels are done only on individual pesticides. No one has tested the infinite number of combinations of pesticides we are all regularly exposed to. For example, up to seven different compounds have been found on individual lettuces. Multiple residues on other foods including apples, pears, carrots, oranges, celery and strawberries are also common, and of course several different foods are usually eaten at any given meal. It all adds up to a cocktail of pesticide residues, the combined toxicity of which is almost completely unknown.

You can reduce your exposure by switching to organic foods, which are produced with very few, if any, pesticides. In order of importance, based on concentration and toxicity of residues commonly found, opt for organic:

1. Meat and dairy products
2. Grains and root vegetables
3. Vegetables and fruit where you eat the skins (e.g. tomatoes and strawberries)
4. Vegetables and fruit you can peel or remove the outer leaves (e.g. oranges and cabbages)

If organic is too expensive, washing fruit and vegetables in water with a dash of ordinary vinegar (e.g. 1 tablespoon per gallon) can help to remove pesticide residues. Sadly washing with water alone has little effect as most pesticides are formulated to resist being washed off by the rain.

Chemical self-defence

In addition to using chemicals to help grow or produce our food, man-made chemicals are also added to foods to make them look and taste better or last longer. Despite regulations to only allow chemicals classified as 'safe' to be used in foods, many have been found to cause adverse reactions. For example, the orange food colouring Tartrazine (or E102) can trigger hyperactivity and asthma in sensitive individuals, while the flavour enhancer monosodium glutamate (MSG or E621) has been linked to brain over-excitation. We also know that some of these chemicals actually leach beneficial nutrients from the body, for example the vital mineral zinc. So our advice is to avoid buying foods that contain E numbers or strange sounding compounds – unless you are clear what they are (see box opposite).

Is your water fit to drink?

Water is not simply H_2O. When you turn on the tap, your water can also contain traces of nitrates, trihalomethanes, lead and aluminium – all anti-nutrients in their own right. In the vast majority of Britain, the levels of these pollutants don't exceed maximum safety limits. In Scotland, about five per cent of water tested exceeds the permissible levels of trihalomethanes, which is a cancer-causing agent created as a by-product of treating water with chlorine or bromine. Concerns over pollutants in water have led many people to switch to bottled or filtered water.

Overall, it is much more important to drink water than avoid tap water for its small levels of anti-nutrients. But if you are a purist and want your water super clean, it is best to fit a water filter on the tap you use for drinking water, or use a jug filter. However, filtering or distilling water removes not only impurities, but also many of the naturally occurring minerals. This again pushes up the need for minerals from food.

Out of the frying pan

What we do to food in the kitchen can alter the balance between nutrients and anti-nutrients. Frying food in oil produces what are known as free radicals – these are highly-reactive chemicals that destroy essential fats and nutrients in food and can also damage your body's cells, increasing the risk of cancer, heart disease and premature ageing.

Cooking anything at very high temperatures – even without oil – can also produce powerful cancer-promoting chemicals. So barbecued, chargrilled or blackened foods are also bad for your health. Even baked goods such as crispbreads and some breakfast cereals can be harmful as they contain a toxic by-product called acrylamide, which is produced when food is cooked at very high temperatures.

The bottom line is: eat more raw food, and steam, steam-fry or bake rather than cooking at high heat (see page 106 for cooking techniques).

Minimise pharmaceutical drugs

Many common medicines are also anti-nutrients. For example, statins lower cholesterol but also deplete a vital antioxidant called co-enzyme Q10. Metformin, the most commonly prescribed anti-diabetes drug, depletes Vitamin B12. Most people simply don't realise the scale of damage that can be done by drugs. Research published in the *British Medical Journal* estimates that more than 10,000 deaths each year are associated with prescription drugs – and that excludes any taken in over-dose. A quarter of these occur from painkillers, which can both damage the gut and the liver. Once damaged, the gut becomes more 'leaky', which then increases allergic sensitivity since undigested food proteins can pass through the gut wall. Antibiotics also increase gut damage and wipe out the healthy bacteria in your gut that manufacture significant amounts of B vitamins.

Of course there are times when we all need to take drugs, but my advice is to use them only when you really need to, and not to take them routinely. If you have an ongoing health problem, address the un-derlying cause rather than masking the symptoms with drugs. Part Two of this book with look in more detail at common underlying causes of ill health.

Genetically engineered food

The long-term consequences on our health and our eco-system of gen-etically modified (GM) foods are still not fully understood. These foods are typically grown from seeds that have been modified in a laboratory to include different genetic coding to what would occur naturally – for example to make corn resistant to certain pests or tomatoes grow to a uniform size or colour.

Initial predictions that GM crops would reduce pesticide use have proved unfounded. A 2008 report by Friends of the Earth found that pes-ticide use on GM crops has actually dramatically increased – by up to 15 times on some crops. The promise of increased yields has also not tran-spired. And there are concerns that GM food could pose a serious health risk, with possible side effects involving antibiotic resistance, the creation of new toxins and unexpected allergic reactions.

The reality is that these health concerns remain largely speculative be-cause no one can predict what the outcome of the introduction of GM food into the food chain will be. No adequate safety tests have been car-ried out and no one is monitoring the impact of GM food on the diets of those countries now selling significant quantities of GM products for human consumption. Far too little is known about genes and DNA to predict what the possible unexpected effects of genetic engineering will be. Of the few studies that have been carried out, one trial conducted at the University of Caen in France found that rats fed GM corn developed signs of liver and kidney toxicity. An earlier trial on human volunteers, commissioned by the UK Food Standards Agency, found that GM material passed out of soya and into the gut bacteria of some participants during digestion. Genetic material isn't supposed to cross over between different species, so this gives rise to concern.

Until more is known and safety – or otherwise – can be proven, my advice is to check labels and avoid any foods containing GM ingredients (in particular, soya). This certainly seems to be the advice British MPs are following – all food served in the House of Commons restaurants has to be GM free.

Summary

Today we are all exposed to so many pollutants and anti-nutrients that can cause ill health and disease. These are in the air we breathe, the food we eat and the water we drink. But you can make some positive changes to your diet and lifestyle to reduce this 'environmental load':

- Filter your drinking water or drink natural mineral water.
- Buy organic as much as possible, especially for fruits and vegetables where you eat the skins.
- Never deep-fry foods – instead steam, bake or steam-fry.
- Minimise your use of medical drugs unless they are the only viable option for treating a health problem. If you get frequent aches or infections, investigate the underlying cause rather than relying on painkillers or antibiotics.
- Read Chapter 11 for more on ridding your body of toxins.

5. Your Basic Health Plan

Now we have reviewed the key components of an optimum nutrition diet, we can bring it all together into a template for how and what to eat (summarised in the box opposite).

Applying the 80/20 rule

Swapping a diet of refined or nutrient-depleted foods for a wholefood nutrient-rich diet brings many benefits – you'll feel a lot better and discover new and tasty foods, for example. But there will be times when you want to indulge in fish and chips or the odd cream cake. The 80/20 rule gives you scope to do this without wrecking all your good work. The idea is that if you ensure 80 per cent of your diet is optimal, you can get away with 20 per cent not being as healthy, without it impacting too negatively on your overall health.

Graze don't gorge

Do you feel guilty snacking between meals? Well there's no need to any more! Research shows that eating more often helps to sustain your energy for longer. That's why I advocate eating breakfast (it really is the most important meal of the day), lunch and supper and having two snacks during the day – one mid morning and one mid afternoon. This helps to balance your 'blood sugar', which means maintaining a steady supply of energy throughout the day. As you'll discover in Chapter 7, this is the best way to eat if you want to have abundant energy and achieve a healthy weight.

In Chapter 13 (page 100), we go into more detail on how this can break down in terms of what to eat for each meal and snack.

Top Ten Daily Diet Tips

1. Eat one handful of fresh seeds or nuts (whole or ground) – or one tablespoon of a cold-pressed seed oil.

2. Eat two servings of beans, lentils, quinoa, tofu (soya), 'seed' vegetables or other vegetable protein – or one small serving of lean meat, fish, cheese or a free-range egg – every day.

3. Eat three or more servings a day of fresh fruit (aim for a mix of colours).

4. Eat four or more servings a day of whole grains such as rice, rye, oats, wholewheat, corn or quinoa as cereal, breads, pasta or pulses.

5. Eat five servings a day of dark green, leafy and root vegetables such as watercress, carrots, sweet potatoes, broccoli, Brussels sprouts, spinach, green beans or peppers, either raw or lightly cooked.

6. Drink six glasses of pure water, diluted fruit juices or herbal tea.

7. Eat oily fish three times a week – or take a fish oil supplement containing EPA, DPA and DHA.

8. Choose whole foods – whole grains, lentils, beans, nuts, seeds, fresh fruit and vegetables, organic if possible.

9. Avoid refined, white and sugary foods and processed foods, particularly those containing artificial additives.

10. Avoid fried, burnt and browned food, hydronated fat and excess animal fat.

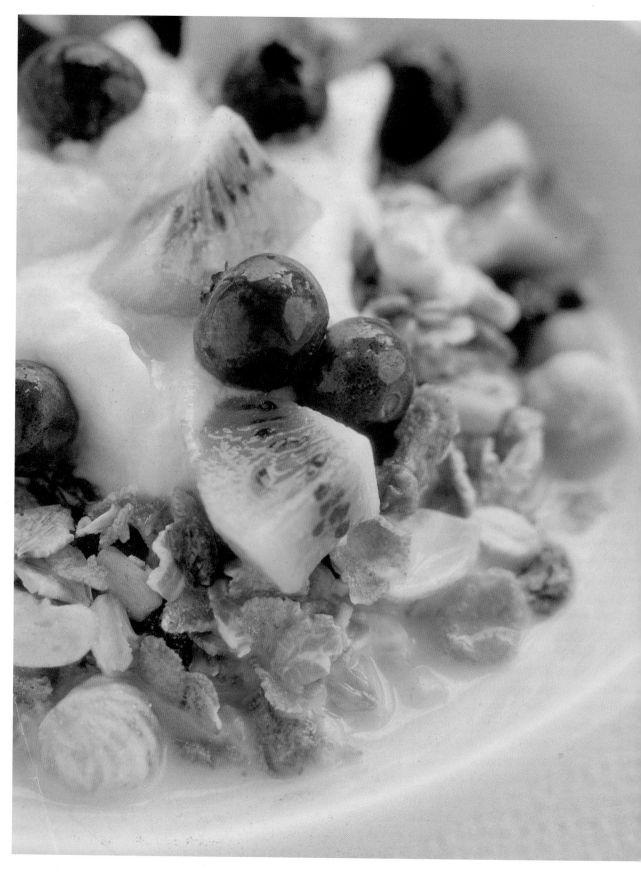

Build your own supplement programme

As we've established in Chapter 3, supplementing your diet with extra vitamins and minerals is essential if you want to achieve your full health potential. We know that the government-set recommended daily allowances (RDAs) are barely adequate, so at the Institute for Optimum Nutrition, we reviewed all the research into the best nutrient levels for optimum health to establish the Optimum Daily Allowances, or ODAs for short (see chart on page 33).

We've calculated the following levels to bridge the shortfall between a good diet (which we outlined earlier) and optimum levels for optimum health (the ODAs). However, we are all different, so the ideal levels for you to supplement will depend not only on the quality of your diet but also on factors such as your age, stress levels, pollution exposure and exercise intensity. As a general rule, these are the sorts of levels to aim for:

Vitamins: Vitamin A 1000mcg, Vitamin C 1–2g, Vitamin D 15mcg, Vitamin E 200mg, Vitamin B1 25mg, Vitamin B2 25mg, Vitamin B3 (also called niacin) 50mg, Vitamin B5 (pantothenic acid) 50mg, Vitamin B6 20mg, Vitamin B12 10mcg, folic acid 200mcg, biotin 50mcg.

Minerals: calcium 200mg, magnesium 150mg, iron 10mg, zinc 10mg, manganese 2.5mg, chromium 30mcg, selenium 50mcg.

Don't worry – it is not necessary to take 19 different supplements every day! Thankfully, you can buy a couple of formulas which contain them all, as follows:

- A multivitamin and mineral with levels of the nutrients outlined above. You can buy formulas which pack all this into one tablet a day – or in two smaller ones, which you take at different times (i.e. one with breakfast and one with lunch or supper).

- Extra Vitamin C – a multivitamin and mineral can't physically fit all the Vitamin C you need each day into just one or two tablets, so you need to take an additional 1000 to 2000mg each day. The best way to take this is in two doses of 500 to 1000mg, preferably at least six hours apart (as Vitamin C doesn't stay in your system any longer than this).

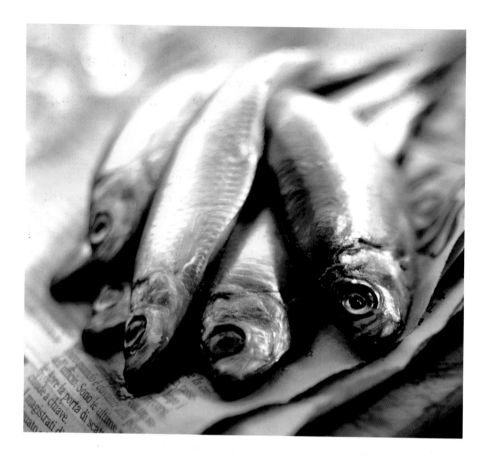

Essential fat supplements

If you eat oily fish three times a week and have some fresh nuts and seeds (or cold-pressed seed oil) every day, then you should be able to source all the essential fats you need from you diet. However, if don't like these foods, have an inflammatory condition (i.e. eczema or asthma – see page 88 for more on this) or have been deficient for a long time, you will need to supplement some Omega 3 and 6 fats as follows:

- Purified fish oils are best for Omega 3 and you need at least 200mg each of the active Omega 3 fats EPA, DPA and DHA, or 600mg of these three combined.

- Starflower oil (also called borage oil) or evening primrose oil are good sources of Omega 6. Starflower oil provides more of the active Omega 6 fat GLA and you need at least 50mg of GLA a day.

So, either supplement one GLA capsule and one fish-oil capsule rich in EPA, DPA and DHA each day, or find a supplement that combines EPA, DPA, DHA and GLA and take two a day.

For all supplements, see the Supplement Directory (page 165) for quality supplement brands I know to be good.

Supplements for specific health problems

On top of a basic supplement programme, you may benefit from taking one or two additional supplements to address a particular health problem and help bring your body back into balance. For example, if you have digestive issues, a 'probiotic' supplement may help (see page 70). Or if you have weight problems, extra chromium may be necessary for a while (see page 56). To help you identify which, if any, could be suitable for you, work your way through the health quizzes in Part Two.

A few important points about supplements

- Take your supplements with food, but avoid taking with coffee or tea, as this can reduce absorption of some vitamins and minerals.

- Do not take individual vitamins or minerals (other than Vitamin C) unless you are also taking a general multi formula – nutrients work together and increasing levels of one without the others can create an imbalance.

- Some supplements are required by law to carry 'advisory notices'. In my view these cautions are, in most cases, exceedingly over-cautious. For example, Vitamin B6 supplements containing above 10mg have to say 'long-term intakes may lead to mild tingling and numbness'. I know of not one single case where this has actually happened, although it can occur at higher doses above 1000mg. However, if you stick to the levels recommended throughout this book, you will stay far below any potentially unsafe levels.

- Lastly, to get the most benefit from your supplements, take them every day. Irregular supplementation doesn't produce the same benefits.

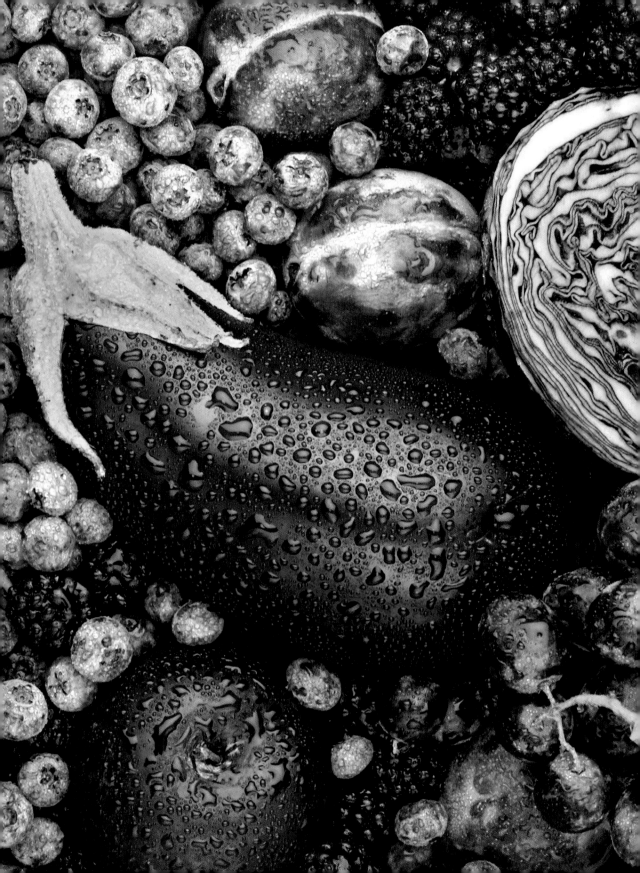

Part Two

Achieving 100% Health

6. Six Steps to Superhealth

There are six key processes that go on inside your body which are core to your overall health. If you are able to maximise how each one functions, then you will be firing on all six cylinders and will feel the benefit in terms of increased energy and well-being and freedom from disease.

Likewise, if you are not functioning well in one area, then it's likely to have a knock-on effect in other areas. For example, if your blood sugar control is poor – and you're gaining weight and feeling low in energy – then the chances are that over time, your hormones will become imbalanced. Your mood and memory are likely to suffer too and you may start to feel a bit down sometimes or find it harder to concentrate. The first stage in stopping – or reversing – this downward spiral, is to identify the areas that are going out of balance. And that's what we'll do in this section of the book.

Over the next six chapters, we will explore each of the six areas in turn. At the start of each chapter, there is a quiz for you to score yourself in that particular area of your health. By the time you've worked your way through all six, you will know which areas need your attention. It may be one or two, or all six!

There are also three levels of priority for each process – red for urgent, yellow for important and green for fine-tuning needed. Doing the quiz and working out your results will help you to determine how you measure up in each of the six areas. In Part Four, you can use the results to prioritise your own personal route to better health.

If you want to share the quizzes with your family or friends – or don't want to mark the book – you can also go online at *www.patrickholford. com* (select 'free online health assessment') for a free assessment of your health, giving you scores for each of these areas.

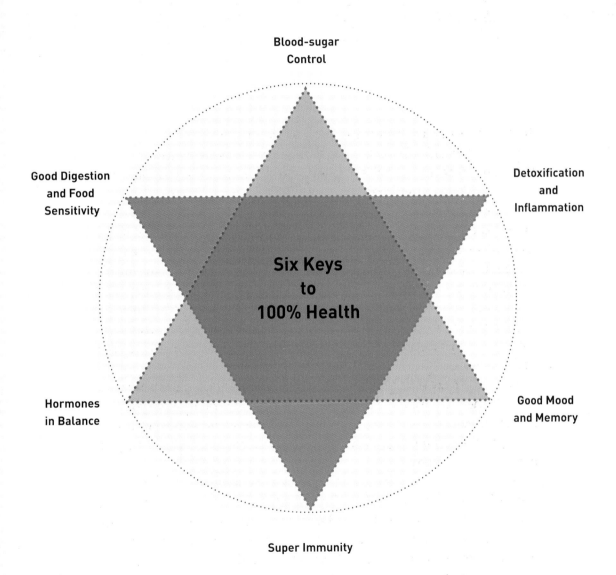

crease Your Energy and Lose Weight

BLOOD SUGAR QUIZ

- [ ] Are you rarely wide awake within 15 minutes of rising?

- [ ] Do you need tea, coffee, a cigarette or something sweet to get you going in the morning?

- [ ] Do you crave chocolate, sweet foods, bread, cereal or pasta?

- [ ] Do you add sugar to your drinks, have sugary drinks or add sugary sauces such as ketchup to your food?

- [ ] Do you often have energy slumps during the day or after meals?

- [ ] Do you crave something sweet or a stimulant after meals?

- [ ] Do you often have mood swings or difficulty concentrating?

- [ ] Do you get dizzy or irritable if you go six hours without food?

- [ ] Do you find you over-react to stress?

- [ ] Is your energy now less than it used to be?

- [ ] Do you feel too tired to exercise?

- [ ] Are you gaining weight, especially on your belly, and finding it hard to lose, even though you're not eating more or exercising less?

How do you score?

0–2 yes answers	3–6 yes answers	More than 7 yes answers
Even a yes to one question in this quiz shows you may have a problem with blood sugar balance – ideally, you want to aim for none! However, you probably only need to fine-tune your existing diet and lifestyle, rather than make radical changes, so read this chapter and introduce the recommendations that don't currently apply to you.	You are starting to show signs of poor blood sugar balance and are no doubt suffering as a result. If you don't address the underlying causes now, you will continue to struggle with maintaining stable energy levels and will probably, if you're not already, start to gain weight. Concentrate on cleaning up your diet and you'll soon start to feel better.	Your blood sugar is seriously imbalanced – but you can reverse the symptoms you are experiencing by following the advice in this chapter. The key challenges for you will be quitting sugary foods and stimulants – but as you cut these out of your diet, you will be rewarded with better energy levels and a more stable weight.

Is your fuel making you tired or fat?

As I explain in Chapter 3, carbohydrate is our fuel of choice – we digest it down into glucose (a type of sugar) and use this to make energy. But in between digestion and making energy, the glucose is absorbed from your digestive tract into your bloodstream. And it's the level in your blood – your blood sugar level – that's key.

Keeping your blood sugar level balanced is probably the most important factor in maintaining stable energy levels and weight. The level of sugar in your blood largely determines your appetite. When the level drops, you feel hungry, so you eat some food. The carbohydrate content of that food is digested down to glucose and this is absorbed into your blood and your blood sugar level rises. Your body then produces a hormone called insulin to take this sugar into your cells to make energy.

However, when you eat food containing too much sugar – i.e. refined and/or sugary carbohydrates such as white bread or biscuits – your blood sugar level rises dramatically. Your body is then unable to take it all into your cells to make energy, so it firstly will convert this sugar into a substance called glycogen and store it in your liver or muscle cells. When your glycogen stores are full, your body will next convert any excess sugar in your blood into fat, your long-term energy reserve. So if you eat a lot of refined and sugary foods, your body will be busy converting the excess sugar they contain to fat, causing you to put on weight.

The other downside of frequent high blood sugar is frequent low blood sugar. This is because your body will clear high sugar levels from your blood very quickly because it's dangerous if left unchecked. Too much sugar makes the blood sticky and can damage arteries and body tissues, which is why diabetics often suffer with nerve and eye damage and leg ulcers. Therefore your body will act fast to correct high blood sugar, and this can often push you from one extreme to the other – you end up with very low blood sugar.

As I've mentioned, when your blood sugar is low, you feel hungry. If you refuel with fast-energy-releasing carbohydrates, you then cause your blood sugar to rise rapidly – and so trigger a repetitive cycle of yo-yoing blood sugar that makes it very hard for you to find a balance and maintain stable blood sugar levels.

The symptoms of low blood sugar include fatigue, poor concentration, irritability, nervousness, sweating, headaches and digestive problems. An estimated three in every ten people have impaired ability to keep their blood sugar level stable. The result, over the years, is that you are likely to become increasingly fat and lethargic. But if you can control your blood sugar levels, the result is even weight and constant energy.

The secret of stable blood sugar

As I've explained, fast-releasing carbohydrates are like rocket fuel, releasing their glucose in a sudden rush. They give a quick burst of energy with

Understanding the Glycemic Load

The Glycemic Load combines the Glycemic Index with the concept of measuring carbohydrate intake to provide a scientifically superior way of controlling blood sugar. Put simply, the Glycemic Index (GI) of a food tells you whether the carbohydrate in the food is fast or slow releasing. It's a 'quality' measure. It doesn't tell you, however, how much of the food is carbohydrate. Carbohydrate points, or grams of carbohydrate, tell you how much of the food is carbohydrate, but it doesn't tell you what the particular carbohydrate does to your blood sugar. It's a 'quantity' measure. The Glycemic Load (GL) of a food is the quantity times the quality. For a complete list of foods and their GL scores, log on to *www.holforddiet.com*.

a rapid burn-out. So if you want to balance your blood sugar, you need to eat less fast-releasing (i.e. cakes, biscuits, sweets) and more slow-releasing foods (wholegrain carbohydrates, fresh fruit and vegetables).

Fast or slow: the GL guide

The best way to achieve stable blood sugar balance is to control the Glycemic Load – or GL for short – of your diet. You may have heard of the 'Glycemic Index' or know about the connection between restricting carbohydrates and weight loss, as pioneered by Atkins. The Glycemic Load develops these concepts to the next stage to create a scientifically superior way of controlling blood sugar (see box opposite).

The reason we focus on the carbohydrate content of foods is because the other two main food types – fat and protein – don't have any appreciable effect on blood sugar. In fact, I recommend you eat some fat and protein with your carbohydrate because this will further lessen the GL score of the carbohydrate you eat.

So for balancing your blood sugar, there are only **three** rules:

Rule 1 Eat 40 GLs a day to lose weight, 60 to maintain it.
Rule 2 Eat carbohydrate with protein.
Rule 3 Graze don't gorge.

The third rule means eating little and often. So always eat breakfast, lunch and supper – and introduce a snack mid morning and mid afternoon. This way you'll provide your body with a constant supply of fuel.

Turn to Chapter 13, page 100 to see how this works in practice.

Breaking the sugar habit

The taste for concentrated sweetness is often acquired in childhood. If sweet things are used as a reward or to cheer someone up, they become emotional comforters. The best way to break the habit is to avoid concentrated sweetness in the form of sugar, sweets, sweet desserts, dried fruit and neat fruit juice. Instead, dilute fruit juice and get used to eating fruit instead of having a dessert. Sweeten breakfast cereals with fruit, and have fruit instead of sweet snacks. If you gradually reduce the sweetness in your food, you will get used to the taste.

Why stimulants and stress are bad news

As far as blood sugar problems are concerned, sugar is only one side of the coin. Stimulants and stress are the other. You see, while eating carbohydrates will raise blood sugar, having an alcoholic drink, a coffee, tea or a cigarette – or getting stressed – will do the same. This is because stimulants and stress trigger the release of a hormone called adrenaline – and adrenaline unlocks your body stores of sugar (called glycogen and stored in your muscles and liver). So even if you don't eat sugary or refined foods, if you regularly consume alcohol, caffeine-containing stimulants (e.g. coffee, tea, cola or chocolate), smoke or are frequently stressed, you will more than likely have imbalanced blood sugar.

Don't be fooled into thinking stimulants give you energy – on the contrary, they do the opposite when you regularly consume them. Research has found that coffee drinkers, for example, don't feel any better than people who never drink coffee – they just feel better than before they had their caffeine fix. In other words, drinking coffee relieves the symptoms of withdrawal from coffee. It's addictive.

The answer, therefore, is to reduce your intake of stimulants – seeking professional help to quit smoking if you need it – and follow the advice to balance your blood sugar by eating a low GL diet. If stress is a problem for you, follow the advice on page 149.

As you teach your body to make energy from your food, you'll need to rely less on using stimulants (or stress) as an energy source.

Additional supplements for blood sugar balance and weight loss

The ability to turn food efficiently into energy instead of fat depends upon hundreds of enzymes which, in turn, depend upon vitamins and minerals. To tune up your metabolism for fat burning, it is essential to consume optimal amounts of these nutrients. In Chapter 5, I recommend a basic supplement programme which provides a good level of all essential nutrients. If your score puts you in the red in this section, or you want to lose weight, there are two additional supplements which can help.

Chromium: This mineral is often lacking in the modern diet – yet it is essential for stablising blood sugar, and therefore energy levels and weight. Chromium is found in wholemeal flour, bread and pasta, as well as in asparagus, mushrooms, beans, nuts and seeds. It works in partnership

Sugar Alternatives

Beware switching to natural sugars such as honey or maple syrup as these still cause a rapid increase in blood sugar. Artificial sweeteners are not so great either. Some have been shown to have harmful effects on health, and all perpetuate a sweet tooth. One of the best sugar alternatives is xylitol, a vegetable sugar that has a very low GL. It tastes much the same as regular sugar but has little effect on blood sugar. Nine teaspoons of xylitol, for example, have the equivalent effect as just one teaspoon of regular sugar or honey.

with Vitamin B3 (also rich in mushrooms and whole wheat, plus salmon, mackerel and turkey). I recommend supplementing 200mcg of chromium a day for a month, plus the equivalent of half a teaspoon of cinnamon if you have blood sugar problems, weight gain or carbohydrate cravings.

Hydroxycitric acid: Although it isn't a vitamin, hydroxycitric acid (HCA) could help you lose weight. Extracted from the dried rind of the tamarind fruit, HCA is proven to slow down the production of fat and reduce appetite, and has no apparent toxicity or safety concerns. In one scientific trial, it generated nearly three times more weight loss in dieters supplementing it, compared to those who weren't. HCA could therefore be a useful addition to a low-GL diet if you're looking to lose weight. It is widely available as a supplement, often found in combination with chromium. If you are interested in using HCA, I recommend taking 750mg a day (see Resources for suppliers). An amino acid called 5-HTP is also effective (see page 96).

Summary

To balance your blood sugar, which will help you achieve stable energy and regulate your weight:

- Choose low-GL foods.
- Eat carbs with an equal amount of protein.
- Graze rather than gorge.
- Avoid refined carbohydrates and sugary foods.
- Avoid caffeine (tea, coffee, caffeinated drinks).
- Don't smoke.
- Minimise alcohol intake.

FIND OUT MORE
Read *The Holford Low-GL Diet Made Easy*, *Holford Low-GL Diet Cookbook* and *Holford Diet GL Counter* (all published by Piatkus).

8. Digestion Perfection

DIGESTIVE HEALTH QUIZ

☐ Do you eat too fast and fail to chew your food thoroughly?

☐ Do you sometimes suffer from bad breath?

☐ Do you often get a burning sensation in your stomach or regularly use indigestion tablets?

☐ Do you often have a feeling of fullness in your stomach?

☐ Do you often get diarrhoea?

☐ Do you often suffer from constipation?

☐ Do you often get a bloated stomach?

☐ Do you often feel nauseous?

☐ Do you often belch or pass wind?

☐ Do you often get stomach pains?

☐ Do you fail to have a bowel movement at least once a day?

☐ Do you feel worse, or excessively sleepy, after meals?

How do you score?

0–3 yes answers	4–7 yes answers	7 or more yes answers
You are unlikely to have a digestive problem, unless you suffer severely from only a couple of symptoms. But for perfect digestion, the ideal score is 0, so you can still improve things by following the advice in this chapter.	You are beginning to show signs of digestive difficulties. Avoiding digestive irritants and concentrating on simple activities such as chewing more thoroughly should be your initial focus.	There's a very good chance that your digestion needs some support. Focus on improving your diet and taking the necessary supplements to repair any damage to your digestive tract.

You are not just what you eat

The popular phrase 'you are what you eat' is only partly true – you are also what you can digest and absorb. Digestion is fundamental to health – and it's an amazing process. Over your lifetime, more than 100 tons of food will pass along your digestive tract. This is a 30-foot long tube – much of it lined with tiny protrusions (like bristles on a brush) – and if you pulled it out and ironed it flat, it would be the size of a small football pitch! The skin that lines this tube is less than paper thin – it's actually a quarter of the thickness of a sheet of paper, so it can become easily damaged. That's why it replaces itself every four days.

Your ability to digest well affects more than just your digestive health – it determines your energy levels, affects your immune system, has a knock-on effect on your mental state, hormonal balance and ability to detoxify. A lack of nutrients, the wrong kind of food, high stress levels and drug and antibiotic use can all impair digestion.

Why chewing is more important than you think

Most of us bolt down our food too fast and are too rushed to take time to really enjoy and chew it thoroughly. Yet this is the first stage on the production line of digestion – get this wrong, and the whole process is affected. Teeth are designed to grind down food into a liquid mush, hence the advice 'drink your food, chew your liquids'. So ideally, aim to chew each mouthful 20 times – yes, really!

Once food has been thoroughly chewed and mixed with saliva (which starts to break down carbohydrate), it passes down the oesophagus into the stomach. Here it is churned up with stomach acid, which disinfects your food to kill off any possible bugs and starts to break down protein and liberate vitamins and minerals for absorption. Your stomach also produces an enzyme called pepsinogen which aids protein digestion.

The production of stomach acid (also called betaine hydrochloride) is dependent on zinc – so if you are deficient, then you probably won't be making enough. Stomach acid production often declines in old age, as do zinc levels. The consequence is indigestion (e.g. burping, flatulence, bloating and a heavy feeling after eating), and an increased likelihood of developing food allergies (see page 63).

Some people produce too much stomach acid and get a burning sensation in the stomach. Avoiding acid-forming and irritating substances can help to alleviate this. Alcohol, coffee, tea and aspirin all irritate the gut wall, while meat, fish, eggs and other concentrated proteins stimulate acid production and can aggravate over-acidity. The minerals calcium and magnesium are particularly alkaline and tend to have a calming effect on people suffering from excess acidity.

Enzymes digest your food

Once the stomach has done its job, your food will pass into your small intestines for further digestion. Here, more enzymes are released (from your pancreas and gallbladder) and these continue to break down protein and carbohydrates and start to break down fats.

Your production of digestive enzymes is critical to trouble-free digestion and absorption. When your body is working optimally, you produce ten litres of these enzymes a day! But adequate production depends on many nutrients, especially Vitamin B6 and zinc. Poor nutrition often results in poor digestion, which in turn creates poor absorption so that nutritional intake gets worse and worse. The consequence is that your food remains undigested and can start to putrify. This can damage your gut lining, making it 'leaky' so that undigested molecules of food can get through into your bloodstream, which can trigger an allergic reaction to everyday foods. It also encourages bad bacteria and other micro-organisms to grow, which can result in you experiencing flatulence, abdominal pain and bloating.

The easiest way to correct this kind of problem is to take a broad-spectrum digestive enzyme supplement with each meal, plus a healing nutrient such as glutamine to help repair any damage to the gut lining.

These usually only need to be taken for a month to get your digestive tract working optimally again.

The friendly bugs in your gut

Did you know that up to four pounds of your body weight comes from bacteria that lives in your digestive tract? The average person has around 100 trillion bacteria, mostly living in the colon. These are a mix of good and bad bacteria – for healthy digestion, the balance needs to be mostly good. The good (or friendly) bacteria perform a number of roles such as:

- **Make vitamins,** including A, K and B, and also improve the absorption of minerals such as calcium and magnesium.

- **Inhibit 'bad' bacteria,** fungi and viruses that can cause infections and food poisoning.

- **Boost your immunity** by increasing the number of immune cells.

- **Repair and promote the health of the digestive tract** by fermenting fibre into fuel for cells in the intestinal lining, helping it to regenerate.

- **Reduce allergic reactions** by helping to keep the digestive tract healthy, so it's less likely the immune system will react to a food.

However, the balance of bacteria can easily be upset – for example, after taking antibiotics, which wipe them out, or having too many sugary and refined foods or alcohol. If bad bacteria then proliferate, you can experience a wide range of symptoms including constipation or diarrhoea, bloating, flatulence, foul-smelling stools, food intolerances, increased infections and skin problems. It is possible to test for different types and levels of gut bacteria via a simple home test (see the Resources section).

If you suspect you have an imbalance in gut bacteria, you can repopulate your digestive tract with good bacteria by taking a 'probiotic' supplement. There are an increasing number of yoghurt probiotic drinks available now, but many of these contain what are called 'transitory' strains of bacteria – this means they may have a beneficial effect as they pass through you, but they are not the resident strains that actually live nside you. They often contain a lot of sugar as well. If you want to increase levels of good bacteria, then you need to supplement the resident strains – the principal families are called Lactobacillus and Bifidus bacteria.

Studies have shown that supplementing probiotics can ease a range of digestive disorders including Crohn's disease, ulcerative colitis, diarrhoea and irritable bowel syndrome. Research suggests that about half of all those diagnosed with irritable bowel syndrome have an abnormal bacteria balance and therefore are likely to benefit from probiotics. Diarrhoea also responds well – probiotics can halve recovery time.

You can also boost your level of beneficial bacteria by eating fermented foods such as live natural yoghurt, miso (the Japanese soya paste used in miso soup) and sauerkraut.

Is your food making you ill?

As many as one in five adults and children has an allergic reaction to everyday foods such as milk, wheat, yeast and eggs – but many simply

Curing Constipation

This is a surprisingly common problem – more than 80 per cent of people fail to have a bowel movement every day. Modern diets often lack fibre and water – two cornerstones for healthy digestion – and are also rich in wheat, which can be abrasive and difficult to digest. Fruit, vegetables and non-wheat wholegrains (particularly oats and brown rice) contain soluble fibres which encourage the smooth and regular passage of waste matter. So switching to an optimum nutrition diet should encourage good digestion, as will drinking 1.5–2 litres of water a day, preferably in between meals. Prunes, figs and kiwi fruit are natural laxatives. Or try stirring a dessertspoon of linseeds into a glass of water before bed and drinking down the gloppy liquid in the morning (you can also add this to smoothies or juices). Taking digestive enzymes and probiotics (see text opposite) can also help, as can supplementing 200mg of magnesium and 1000mg of Vitamin C two to three times a day. And finally, exercise is essential for good digestion, especially if you stimulate the abdominal area. It also relieves stress, which can impact negatively on digestion.

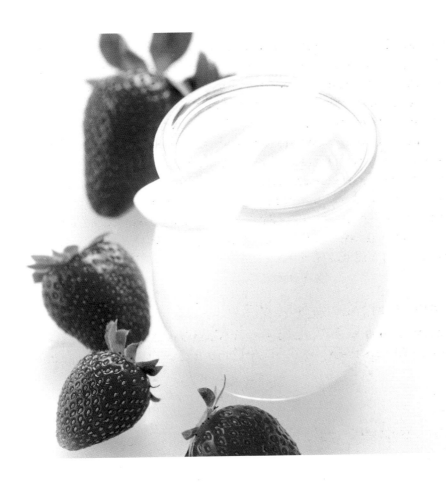

don't know it. Yet these reactions can cause a diverse range of seemingly unconnected symptoms – from fatigue to depression; digestive problems to headaches. If you can tick 'yes' to four or more of the questions on the following page, consider food allergy as a potential culprit.

Not all allergies are the same

Most people are familiar with what's called 'classical' food allergy. This is usually an immediate and severe reaction to a food – such as peanuts or seafood – that may be life threatening. If you have this type of allergy, you probably already know about it and are strictly avoiding the offending food. But the most common food allergies can take from one hour to three days to emerge and the reaction is less dramatic and therefore harder to detect. These are often called 'hidden' food allergies. Both kinds of allergy

FOOD SENSITIVITY QUIZ

[ ] Can you gain weight in hours?

[ ] Do you get bloated after eating?

[ ] Do you suffer from diarrhoea or constipation?

[ ] Do you suffer from abdominal pain?

[ ] Do you sometimes get really sleepy after eating?

[ ] Do you suffer from headaches?

[ ] Do you suffer from rashes, itches, asthma or shortness of breath?

[ ] Do you have dark circles under the eyes or puffy eyes?

[ ] Do you suffer from other aches or pains?

[ ] Do you get better on holidays abroad, when your diet is completely different?

How do you score?

involve the immune system, but trigger a different type of reaction.

A third kind of reaction to food doesn't involve the immune system at all. This is often called an 'intolerance'. For example, lactose intolerance is where a person lacks the enzyme to digest the sugar in dairy products (lactose), usually resulting in digestive symptoms such as diarrhoea and abdominal pains. This can be bypassed by supplementing the 'lactase' enzyme (see Supplement Directory).

Testing for allergies

If you suspect you might have an allergy, you can arrange for an allergy test. The best test, called an 'IgG ELISA' test, uses a finger-prick blood sample and is available as a home-test kit (see Resources). Alternatively, you can try an elimination-and-challenge diet. This involves removing any likely culprits from your diet for a two-week minimum period and noting any changes in physical or mental symptoms. Then you reintroduce the foods one at a time, leaving 24 hours in between, and you closely monitor your reaction. For either, testing is best done under the guidance of a nutritional therapist or allergy expert who can support you and devise a suitable diet to compensate for the subsequent removal of any allergenic foods.

The good news is that 'hidden' allergens do not need to be avoided for ever (sadly, classical allergens often do). If you strictly avoid the food(s) you've identified and improve your overall digestive health – by eating an optimum nutrition diet, supplementing digestive enzymes and probiotics and healing the gut with nutrients such as glutamine – you can often reintroduce them with no reaction after four months.

Summary

Good digestion is essential to good health, yet digestive problems are surprisingly common. To improve your digestion:

- Eat an optimum nutrition diet.
- Minimise wheat and increase beneficial fibres from oats, rice, fruits and vegetables.
- Drink 1.5–2 litres of liquid as water or herb teas, between meals.
- Eat live, natural, organic yoghurt (soya or dairy) twice a week.
- Sit down, relax and take your time over your meals.
- Chew your food thoroughly.

If you have digestive problems, in addition to the above, aim to:
- Find out and avoid what you are allergic to.
- Take a broad-spectrum digestive enzyme to improve absorption.
- If you suffer with acid stomach after eating, avoid acid-forming and irritating foods and drinks, and investigate food allergies.
- Take a teaspoon of glutamine powder, last thing at night in water, to help heal any damage to your gut lining.
- Take a daily probiotic supplement containing Lactobacillus acidophilus and Bifidobacteria (see Supplement Directory).

FIND OUT MORE
Read *Improve Your Digestion*, by Patrick Holford, and *Hidden Food Allergies*, by Patrick Holford and Dr James Braly (published by Piatkus).

9. Boost Your Immune System

IMMUNE SYSTEM QUIZ

- [ ] Do you get more than three colds a year?

- [ ] Do you usually get a stomach bug each year?

- [ ] Do you find it hard to shift an infection (cold or otherwise)?

- [ ] Are you prone to thrush or cystitis?

- [ ] Do you generally take at least one course of antibiotics each year?

- [ ] Has more than one member of your immediate family had cancer?

- [ ] Do the glands in your neck, armpits or groin feel tender?

- [ ] Do you suffer from allergy problems?

- [ ] Do you have an inflammatory disease such as eczema, asthma or arthritis?

- [ ] Do you often have a stuffy or runny nose, or suffer with hayfever?

- [ ] Do you have an autoimmune disease such as rheumatoid arthritis or lupus?

- [ ] Have you been diagnosed with cancer or pre-cancerous growths?

How do you score?

0–3 yes answers	4–6 yes answers	More than 7 yes answers
So few symptoms suggests that your immune system is quite strong. Focus on the preventative measures to ensure you continue to be healthy, and support your immune system to ensure you don't succumb to illness.	You are starting to show signs of reduced immunity. Following an optimum nutrition approach will certainly help to support your immune system, but also focus on prevention too.	Your immune system is in real need of support. Cleaning up your diet will remove many immune suppressants – but focus too on others highlighted here, and give yourself a boost by increasing the immune-supporting nutrients.

Increase immunity from inside

When you are younger, it is easy to fool yourself into believing that all those degenerative and life-threatening diseases will only happen to other people. But are you really immune to both minor and major infections, and will cancer pass you by? Are you free from allergies and do you rarely suffer from a cold? If you want to answer yes, then you're on the right track.

For the past 100 years, medicine has focused on drugs designed to destroy the invader – antibiotics, anti-viral agents, chemotherapy. While sometimes necessary, these drugs can harm the body. For example, antibiotics can damage the digestive tract and upset the balance of beneficial bacteria, leading to secondary infections such as thrush. Overuse of antibiotics is also encouraging the evolution of new drug-resistant strains of bacteria which can be deadly for vulnerable people.

Only recently, with the seemingly endless onslaught of new infectious agents, has attention turned within – towards strengthening the body, rather than conquering the invading organism. The immune system is one of the most remarkable and complex systems within the human body. When you realise that it has the ability to produce a million antibodies within a minute and to recognise and disarm a billion different invaders, the strategy of boosting immune power makes a lot of sense. The ability to react rapidly to a new invader makes all the difference between a minor 24-hour cold or a week in bed with flu. It may also be the difference between a non-malignant lump and breast cancer, or a minor or major infection.

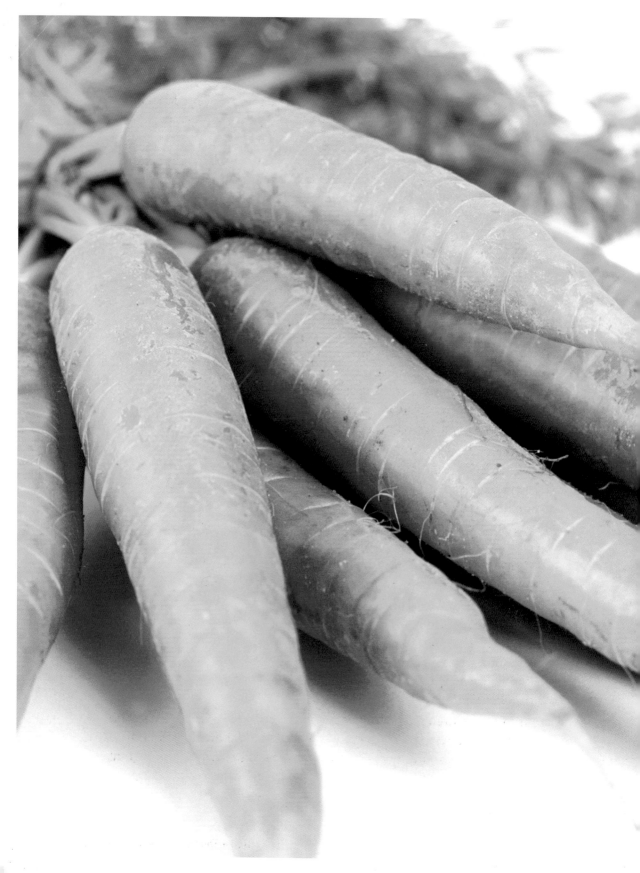

How do you boost your immune system? Exercise, your state of mind and your diet all play a part. Over-training actually suppresses the immune system, while calming exercise such as yoga or t'ai chi can stimulate it. Stress and grief also depress the immune system, so learning how to cope with stress, dealing with psychological issues and relaxing regularly is an important part of boosting the immune system. Meditation, for example, has been shown to increase immune cell counts.

The immune power diet

The ideal immune-boosting diet is, in essence, no different from the ideal diet for anyone. Since immune cells are produced rapidly during an infection, sufficient protein is essential. Eating the right kinds of fats is important too. Diets high in saturated or hydrogenated fat suppress immunity and clog up the system, while essential fats – found in oily fish, nuts and seeds – boost immune function.

If you have an infection that increases mucus production (e.g. a cold), it is best to avoid dairy produce – this tend to stimulate more mucus.

To ensure you get plenty of immune-boosting nutrients, eat plenty of fresh fruit and vegetables. Good sources include carrots, beetroot, sweet potatoes, tomatoes and beansprouts, plus watermelon and berries (strawberries, blueberries, raspberries, etc – you can buy these frozen when they are not in season). Eat what you can raw, and lightly steam the rest. Avoid frying anything as this introduces harmful free radicals that increase your toxic load (see page 38).

Sugar is not good news at the best of times, but studies show that it can actually depress immune activity, so avoid any forms if you are fighting an infection. Also avoid refined grains (which quickly digest down to sugar and contain few nutrients), instead opting for wholegrains (oats, rye bread, brown rice, etc).

Immune-boosting nutrients

Your immune strength is totally dependent on an optimal intake of vitamins and minerals. Deficiency of Vitamins A, B1, B2, B6, B12, folic acid, C and E suppress immunity, as does insufficient iron, zinc, magnesium and selenium.

Since no nutrients work in isolation, it is a good idea to take a good high-strength multivitamin and mineral supplement. Scientific studies have demonstrated that the combination of nutrients at even modest levels can boost immunity very effectively.

Antioxidant action

The nutrients worth adding in larger amounts to fight off infections are the antioxidants, and particularly Vitamin C. These work together to help weaken any invader. For example, Vitamin A helps to maintain the integrity of the digestive tract, lungs and all cell membranes, preventing foreign agents from entering the body and viruses from entering cells. Vitamin E and selenium improve immune cell function, and zinc is especially important as it is crucial for immune cell production.

Vitamin C is unquestionably the master immune-boosting nutrient. As well as supporting immune cell production and function, it has both anti-viral and anti-bacterial actions and can reduce inflammation. However, it is needed in quite high doses to do its job effectively – see box, How to Kill a Cold.

Probiotics – nature's antibiotics

Infectious agents are all around us. Whether or not you succumb to them is determined not only by your exposure, but also by the balance of beneficial bacteria in your body. As we explored in Chapter 8, you have pounds

How to Kill a Cold

Vitamin C is one of the immune system's most powerful weapons – you just need to ensure the dose is high enough. Based on scientific evidence, the optimum daily dose for cold prevention appears to be 1–2 grams a day. But once you have a cold, much higher levels are needed. This is because you want to 'saturate' your body tissues, which ensures a cold virus isn't able to survive. To do this, you need to take 1 gram an hour. Fortunately, Vitamin C is one of the least toxic substances known to man. The only side effect you may experience is loose bowels – if this happens, just reduce the dose 1 gram every two hours until the cold had gone.

Immune Power Soup

This recipe includes seven anti-inflammatory and immune-boosting foods. The quantities aren't exact – in fact, you can play around with them to suit your taste.

1. Chop up two large red onions and crush four garlic cloves and sauté in a little coconut oil, but don't brown.

2. Chop up six carrots and three sweet potatoes or a butternut squash into pieces about half an inch square. Add to the onions and garlic and pour in enough boiling water to just cover.

3. Add in loads of fresh chopped ginger, a teaspoon of turmeric and about a quarter teaspoon of cayenne (to taste). These are powerful infection fighters.

4. Bring the soup to the boil and simmer for about 15 minutes, or until the carrots and sweet potato/squash are soft.

5. Add in a diced red pepper, high in vitamin C, and half a cup of coconut milk and purée to a thick soup consistency and serve with oatcakes or pumpernickel.

of bacteria in your digestive tract – as long as the balance is mostly good, these help to inhibit bad bacteria from causing infections. If not kept in check, Salmonella, for example, can cause food poisoning, while Staphylococci can cause sore throats and Candida Albicans thrush.

You can boost your level of beneficial bacteria by taking a probiotic supplement. These are nature's antibiotics and as well as helping you inhibit the bad bacteria that cause illness, research has found they also improve the fighting power of your immune system. Along with providing general immune support, probiotics are proven helpful in treating thrush, recurrent bladder infections, sinusitis and tonsillitis.

Immune-boosting herbs

Herbs can be a useful addition to the natural medicine cupboard. Six excellent ones are:

Cat's claw: A powerful anti-viral, antioxidant and immune-boosting agent from the Peruvian rainforest, cat's claw is available in supplements or as a tea. Dose when fighting an infection: 2–6 grams a day, or 2–6 cups of tea.

Echinacea: This great all-rounder has anti-viral and anti-bacterial properties. It comes in capsules or as a tincture. Dose when fighting an infection: 2–3 grams a day, or 15 drops three times a day.

Black elderberry extract: Reduces the duration of colds and flu by preventing the virus from taking hold. Dose when fighting an infection: 1 dessertspoon three times a day.

Garlic: Anti-viral, anti-fungal and anti-bacterial. Include a clove a day in your daily diet. For infections, increase to 2–6 cloves a day (or take it in supplementary form).

Ginger: Particularly good for sore throats and stomach upsets. Put six slices of fresh root ginger in a thermos with a stick of cinnamon and fill up with boiling water – five minutes later you have a delicious, throat-

Immune superfoods

Watermelon – the flesh is rich in Vitamins A and C and the seeds are a good source of zinc, selenium, Vitamin E and essential fats. Blend together the flesh and seeds to make a delicious juice and drink a pint for breakfast and another pint during the day.

Carrots – provide a rich source of betacarotene. Other orange vegetables also provide this immune-boosting nutrient, such as sweet potatoes, apricots and butternut squash.

Seed vegetables – these contain antioxidant nutrients plus protein. Make a large salad with broad beans, broccoli, grated carrot, beetroot, courgettes, watercress, lettuce, tomatoes and avocados, adding seeds or marinated tofu pieces – organic if possible. Serve with a dressing of cold-pressed oil containing some crushed garlic.

Berries – strawberries have more Vitamin C than oranges, and blueberries have the highest antioxidant power score of all. Raspberries and strawberries are also excellent and, like all berries, contain many phytonutrients that boost your immune system. So, when you are under attack, snack on berries – the more the merrier.

soothing ginger and cinnamon tea. You can add a little lemon and honey for taste.

Grapefruit seed extract: A powerful natural antibiotic, anti-fungal and anti-viral agent, grapefruit seed extract comes in drops and can be swallowed, gargled or used as nose or ear drops, depending on the site of infection. Dose when fighting an infection: 20–30 drops a day.

Summary

Your immune system needs the right nutrients to function effectively. Following the optimum nutrition diet outlined in Chapter 5 will help you provide a daily intake of these, while also limiting foods which suppress the immune system, such as refined sugar.

In addition, to support healthy immunity on an ongoing basis:
- Do some regular gentle exercise such as t'ai chi or yoga.
- Learn to handle stress and relax daily.
- Take a high-strength multivitamin and mineral supplement, plus an extra 1–2g of Vitamin C.
- Take an antioxidant formula that provides at least 1500mcg of Vitamin A, 200mg of Vitamin E, 10mg of zinc and 50mcg of selenium.

If you are fighting an infection, in addition to the above, try the following:
- Eat lightly, making sure you get enough protein, which is needed to build immune cells. If you have a mucus-related infection, avoid dairy products.
- Take extra Vitamin C – 3 grams every four hours (if it has a laxative effect, reduce the dose slightly).
- Take a daily probiotic supplement (see Supplement Directory).
- If you have a cold, take one dessertspoon of black elderberry extract four times a day.
- Drink cat's claw tea and consider adding ginger and echinacea drops.
- Eat more garlic, or take garlic capsules.
- Find out what your infection is and, if necessary, see your doctor, especially if you are not better within five days.

FIND OUT MORE
Read *Boost your Immune System* by Patrick Holford and Jennifer Meek (published by Piatkus).

10. Balancing Hormones Naturally

FEMALE HORMONE BALANCE QUIZ

☐ Do you use the contraceptive pill or HRT, or have you been on either for more than three years in the last seven years?

☐ Do you experience cyclical water retention, mood swings or depression?

☐ Do you have excess hair on your body or thinning hair on your scalp?

☐ Have you gained weight on your thighs and hips?

☐ Have you at any time been bothered with problems affecting your reproductive organs (ovaries or womb)?

☐ Do you have fertility problems, difficulty conceiving or a history of miscarriage?

☐ Are your periods often painful, irregular or heavy?

☐ Do you suffer from lumpy or tender breasts?

☐ Do you suffer from reduced libido or loss of interest in sex?

☐ Do you suffer from anxiety, panic attacks or nervousness?

☐ Do you suffer from hot flushes or vaginal pain or dryness?

How do you score?

MALE HORMONE BALANCE QUIZ

☐ Are you gaining weight?

☐ Do you often suffer from mood swings or depression?

☐ Have you at any time been bothered with problems affecting your reproductive organs (prostate or testes)?

☐ Do you suffer from reduced libido or loss of interest in sex?

☐ Do you suffer from impotence?

☐ Do you have fewer morning erections or have difficulty maintaining an erection?

☐ Do you suffer from fatigue or loss of energy?

☐ Do you suffer from irritability or anger?

☐ Have you had a drop in your motivation and drive?

☐ Do you feel that you are ageing prematurely?

☐ Do you easily become stressed?

☐ Do you have night sweats or suffer from excessive sweating?

How do you score?

0–3 yes answers	4–6 yes answers	More than 7 yes answers
You are unlikely to have a hormone imbalance unless you have problems with libido, impotence, reduced potency or hot flushes. To be in perfect balance, however, the ideal score is 0, so focus on areas that you can improve.	You are starting to show signs of hormone imbalance. Tune up your weak areas to bring yourself back into balance and eliminate any problems.	Your hormones appear to be out of balance and in need of support. Focus on the diet and supplement suggestions that apply to you, and pursue strategies to learn to deal better with stress if this is an issue for you.

The body's communicators

Some of the most powerful chemicals in the body are hormones – they are your body's communicators. These are produced in special glands and, when released into the bloodstream, give instructions to body cells. Oestrogen, for example, is produced by the ovaries and tells cells to grow – e.g. in the womb lining prior to ovulation, or in breast tissue during pregnancy.

Hormones are made from the food you eat – some, like insulin, from protein; and others, like sex hormones, from cholesterol (despite bad press, this fatty substance is actually important for good health). Any imbalance can have an effect on your overall health.

Thyroid: controlling metabolism

The thyroid gland produces a hormone called thyroxine which controls your metabolism – the rate at which you burn the fuel from your food to make energy and also heat. That's why if you have an over-active thyroid, you can feel wired and be very slim; while if your thyroid is under-active, you can feel tired and be putting on weight.

Having an under-active thyroid is more common and other symptoms include hair loss, constipation and feeling cold. You can test your thyroid function by taking your temperature in the morning – the normal range is 36.5–36.7°C (for women, test in the first half of your menstrual cycle as body temperature increases after ovulation). If you are outside this range, your thyroid may warrant some attention.

In most people, low thyroid function is due to not producing enough thyroxine – often caused by nutrient deficiencies or high stress. It can also be because your immune system is malfunctioning and starts to attack your own thyroid gland. This is why it's important to get a blood test to check for 'thyroid antibodies'. Food allergies, particularly to gluten, can be the trigger, so do check for these too.

Thyroxine is made from an amino acid called tyrosine and is supported by iodine, zinc and selenium. Supplementing these nutrients supports healthy thyroid function. Choose a high-strength multivitamin and mineral supplement that provides these nutrients.

Stress hormones

Your body produces hormones which help you adapt to stress – these are made by your adrenal glands, which sit on top of your kidneys. You are probably familiar with adrenaline, but you also produce hormones called cortisol and DHEA. All three of these hormones work together to help us respond to stressful or emergency situations by channelling the body's energy towards being able to 'fight or take flight', improving oxygen and glucose supply to muscles and generating mental and physical energy. It is a design that helped our ancestors cope with truly life-threatening situations.

In modern life, however, we perceive stress on a much greater scale: for example, when you open your bank statement to find you are overdrawn or get stuck in a traffic jam. Tea, coffee, chocolate and cigarettes have the same effect as they contain stimulants (e.g. caffeine or nicotine) which trigger the release of adrenaline. This results in a burst of energy – but over time, there's a downside. The body slows down digestion, repair and maintenance to channel energy into dealing with stress. As a consequence, prolonged stress is associated with speeding up the ageing process, increasing risk of disease and upsetting overall hormone balance. When your thyroid suffers, for example, your metabolism slows down and you gain weight. Disrupting stress hormones can lead to reduced libido, infertility and menopausal problems.

Get Stress Under Control

Prolonged stress negatively impacts all areas of health. It's therefore important to get it under control by reviewing and eliminating excess sources of stress in your life, or seeking ways to cope better by, for example, doing some daily deep breathing or learning to meditate. Reducing your intake of sugar and stimulants will also help, as will eating an optimum nutrition diet that balances your blood sugar. B vitamins and Vitamin C are important for increasing your resilience to stress so during difficult times, in addition to your daily multivitamin, take 2g of C plus a B complex each day. Magnesium is often called nature's tranquilliser, so taking 200mg twice a day can be calming.

Sex hormones

In women, the two main hormones that control sexual health and reproduction are called oestrogen and progesterone. The balance between these is critical. A relative excess of oestrogen, called 'oestrogen dominance', is associated with an increased risk of breast cancer, fibroids, ovarian cysts and endometriosis. The early warning symptoms of oestrogen dominance include premenstrual syndrome (PMS), depression, loss of sex drive, sweet cravings, heavy periods, weight gain, breast swelling and water retention.

Oestrogen dominance can be due to excess exposure to oestrogenic substances, or a lack of progesterone, or a combination of both. Oestrogenic compounds are found in meat, much of which is hormone fed, in dairy products, in many pesticides and in soft plastics, some of which leach into food when used for wrapping. Oestrogen is also contained in most birth control pills and HRT. So limiting all these sources is important, as is increasing fibre in the diet, which helps to 'escort' excess oestrogen out of the body. Increasing your intake of soya (e.g. tofu), pulses (lentils and hummus) and linseeds can also help to balance hormones.

In both women and men, high stress levels can upset sex hormone balance. Deficiencies of the vitamins and minerals that are needed to make and regulate hormones is very common – in particular Vitamin C, B6, zinc and magnesium. And not getting enough essential fats is another factor – these are needed to make substances which help sensitise cells to hormones.

Beating PMS

Premenstrual syndrome (PMS) affects different women in different ways but usually occurs during the week leading up to a period and includes symptoms such as anxiety, irritability, fluid retention, mood swings, bloating, breast tenderness, weight gain, acne, fatigue, sweet cravings, forgetfulness, headaches and depression.

There are different types of PMS, so finding which one applies to you will help you identify the right nutritional strategy:

- PMS associated with high oestrogen and low progesterone levels – symptoms of which can be bloating, mood swings, fluid retention and breast tenderness. To help reduce oestrogen levels, increase fibre in your diet, eat organically grown produce, reduce meat and dairy consumption and limit your exposure to hormone-disrupting compounds (see page 36).

- PMS associated with food cravings – balancing your blood sugar by following the advice in Chapter 7 will help to reduce cravings, as will boosting your intake of magnesium, chromium and essential fats.

- PMS associated with water retention – magnesium and Vitamin B6 have been shown to be helpful. Reducing your salt intake and increasing water consumption can also reduce water retention.

Managing the menopause

As more evidence gathers on the dangers of HRT, women are increasingly seeking natural alternatives to help them through this stage of life. Symptoms of menopause include hot flushes, irregular periods, vaginal dryness, joint pains, insomnia, headaches and depression. Thankfully, there is a nutritional or herbal solution for most.

Balance your blood sugar – when your blood sugar is not balanced, you are more likely to experience fatigue, irritability, depression and hot flushes. Eating an optimum nutrition diet, balancing low-GL carbs and protein, is the best way to do this (see Chapter 7).

Boost your intake of Vitamin C and E – Vitamin C actually helps your hormones to work, so when levels are low, 1 or 2 grams of Vitamin C (especially a source rich in bioflavonoids) a day can help. Vitamin E is another all-round hormonal helper. A daily intake of 600mg can help vaginal dryness but it takes at least a month to work.

Eat more soya – consuming soya (e.g. as tofu, soya milk or in miso soup) regularly can help to ease hot flushes. Aim to have some every other day.

Up your intake of essential fats – while there isn't much research on the therapeutic effects of essential fats on menopause, they are so vital for balancing hormones that I recommend eating seeds (flax, sunflower and pumpkin) daily and supplementing 500mg of EPA/DPA/DHA and 100mg of GLA.

Agnus Castus – this herb, also called Vitex or Chastetree berry, is a potent hormone balancer that is particularly effective at reducing hot flushes and other menopausal symptoms. The recommended dose is 20–40mg a day.

Men Can Have a Menopause Too

As men get older, testosterone levels drop and some men can experience a 'male menopause' – also known as the andropause. Symptoms include fatigue, depression, decreased sexual performance, redistribution and gain in weight. Following an optimum nutrition diet and supplement programme will help, especially limiting sources of environmental oestrogens (see page 36) which can disrupt male hormone balance. Taking a supplement which supports testosterone production is also useful – look for a formula which contains zinc, Vitamin E and the herbs ginseng, saw palmetto and pygeum.

Physical activity – vigorous exercise has been shown to reduce hot flushes, and yoga can ease menopausal symptoms.

Maximising fertility

One in every four couples suffers from some degree of infertility. While fertility treatment such as IVF is starting to be more widely offered on the NHS, the chances of success are only about 21 per cent. The good news is that an optimum nutrition approach – where any health issues in both the man and the woman are identified and addressed via a personalised nutrition programme – has a 78 per cent success rate. It also results in healthier pregnancies and healthier babies.

Successful conception depends on many factors, some psychological, some physical and some nutritional. Reducing stress and following an optimum nutrition diet and supplement programme is a good start. Both men and women need zinc, Vitamin B6 and essential fats to mature a healthy egg or make high-quality sperm. For men, the mineral chromium can also increase sperm count. Boosting intake of antioxidant nutrients can protect against possible genetic defects in the egg or sperm, and in men, Vitamin C especially can increase sperm count and quality. (See Nutrient Fact Files for food sources of all these nutrients.)

As well as increasing beneficial nutrients, avoiding anti-nutrients is key. These include alcohol, caffeine, tobacco, drugs and exposure to chemicals, either at home or work – studies have shown that these can all decrease fertility in both sexes.

Summary

Hormones are all interrelated, so to ensure yours are balanced, work on promoting optimum function in each key area – thyroid, stress and sex hormones.

- Test your thyroid via a temperature test and supplement tyrosine, iodine, zinc and selenium if it's sluggish (see Supplement Directory for recommended formulas). Also see your GP for a blood test.
- Limit stimulants such as coffee, tea, chocolate, sugar and cigarettes.
- Do not let stress become a habit in your life. Identify sources of stress and make some positive changes to your circumstances and the way you react to them.
- Keep animal fats very low in your diet and eat more soya, pulses and seeds.
- Choose organic vegetables and meat wherever possible to reduce pesticide and hormone exposure.
- Don't eat fatty foods that have been wrapped in cling film (use greaseproof paper instead).
- Make sure you are getting enough essential fats from seeds, their oils or supplements of evening primrose or borage oil (Omega 6) and fish oil (Omega 3).
- Make sure your supplement programme includes optimal levels of Vitamins B3 and B6, magnesium and zinc.
- If you have PMS or menopausal symptoms consider supplementing a hormone-friendly supplement or herbs (see Supplement Directory).
- If you have andropause symptoms or prostate problems supplement saw palmetto and pygeum.

FIND OUT MORE

Read *Balancing Hormones Naturally*, by Patrick Holford and Kate Neil. For help dealing with stress, read *Beat Stress and Fatigue* by Patrick Holford (both Piatkus).

11. Detox and Reduce Inflammation

DETOXIFICATION QUIZ

☐ Do you often suffer from headaches or migraine?

☐ Do you sometimes have watery or itchy eyes or swollen, red or sticky eyelids?

☐ Do you have dark circles under your eyes?

☐ Do you sometimes have itchy ears, earache, ear infections, drainage from the ears or ringing in the ears?

☐ Do you often suffer from excessive mucus, a stuffy nose or sinus problems?

☐ Do you suffer from acne, skin rashes or hives?

☐ Do you sweat a lot and have a strong body odour?

☐ Do you sometimes have joint or muscle aches or pains?

☐ Do you find it hard to lose weight?

☐ Do you often suffer from frequent or urgent urination?

☐ Do you suffer from nausea or vomiting?

☐ Do you often have a bitter taste in your mouth or a furry tongue?

☐ Do you have a strong reaction to alcohol?

☐ Do you suffer from bloating?

☐ Does coffee leave you feeling jittery or unwell?

How do you score?

0–3 yes answers	4–6 yes answers	7 or more yes answers
You are unlikely to have a major problem with detoxification, but could none the less benefit from a short detox to spring-clean your body.	You are beginning to show signs of poor detoxification and need to improve your detox potential by cleaning up your diet.	Your body is complaining – you could seriously benefit from improving your detox potential and eliminating sources of toxins in your daily life.

Detoxification is essential to health

If eating the right food is one side of the optimum health coin, supporting detoxification is the other. As the main organ of detoxification, a well-functioning liver is essential if you want to feel well, look good and slow down the rate at which you age. Just about any allergic, inflammatory or metabolic disorder can be caused by or result from impaired liver function – this includes eczema, asthma, chronic fatigue, recurring infections, inflammatory bowel disorders, multiple sclerosis, rheumatoid arthritis and hormone imbalances. The brain can also be affected if the liver isn't detoxifying effectively – autism, schizophrenia, anxiety, depression and memory loss are all associated with poor liver function.

The good news is that with a good diet, lifestyle and supplements, you can restore and maintain optimal liver function. (There's a simple home test to find out if your liver function is up to scratch – see Resources).

How the body detoxifies

From a chemical perspective, much of what goes on in the body involves substances being broken down, built up and turned from one thing into another. A good 80 per cent of this involves detoxifying potentially harmful substances. Much of this is done by the liver, which represents a clearinghouse able to recognise millions of toxic chemicals and transform them into something harmless or prepare them for elimination. It is the chemical brain of the body – recycling, regenerating and detoxifying in order to maintain your health.

As well as dealing with toxins from the food you eat or air your breathe, your liver has many more to process from all the essential functions that go on inside your body – making energy, digesting food and rebuilding tissues all generate toxins, for example.

Disarming toxins

The liver detoxifies substances by reformatting them so that they become harmless. This process is called conjugation and it requires an adequate supply of nutrients to work effectively. These include antioxidants such as Vitamin A, C and E; foods which contain sulphur, such as onions, garlic and leeks; and cruciferous vegetables (broccoli, cauliflower, kale, cabbage and Brussels sprouts) which contain a family of nutrients called glucosinolates. It's also important to ensure the body isn't too acid, otherwise it can't detoxify as well, so eating plenty of fresh fruit and vegetables will provide alkaline minerals as well as antioxidant nutrients.

WHAT'S YOUR TOXIC LOAD?

☐ Is more than half the food you eat not organic?

☐ Do you spend an hour or more a day in traffic?

☐ Do you live in a city?

☐ Do you smoke, or live with smokers?

☐ Do you often eat fried food?

☐ Do you eat non-organic meat or fish or large fish like tuna or swordfish?

☐ Is most of the food you eat or drink in contact with soft plastic or cling film?

☐ Do you take more than twenty painkillers in a year?

☐ Do you take at least one course of antibiotics each year?

☐ Do have an alcoholic drink on most days?

Score 1 point for each 'yes' answer

The ideal score is 0. A score of 5 or more means you are likely to be taking in a significant quantity of toxins. Any 'yes' answer highlights areas in your diet and lifestyle that warrant attention. To counteract those you can't avoid (e.g. living in a city), ensure you have an adequate intake of detox supplements (see opposite).

Substances that interfere with proper liver function include caffeine, alcohol, recreational and medicinal drugs, the Pill and HRT, industrial pollutants, cigarette smoke, exhaust fumes, high-protein diets, fertilisers on the food we eat, paint fumes, saturated fat, steroid hormones and charcoal-barbecued meat or fish. Needless to say, you should try to avoid any of these that you can and minimise your exposure to the rest.

Detox supplements

It is wise to make sure that your daily supplement programme contains significant quantities of detoxifying antioxidants, especially if you are older, live in a polluted city or have any other unavoidable exposure to oxidants (and also while following any detox regime). The easiest way to do this is by taking a comprehensive antioxidant supplement, in addition to a good multivitamin and mineral. Most reputable supplement companies produce formulas containing a combination of the following nutrients. The kind of total supplementary intake (which may come in part from a multivitamin and extra Vitamin C) to aim for is:

Vitamin A (retinol/betacarotene)	1000mcgRE (3333iu) to 6000mcgRE (20000iu)
Glutathione (reduced) or NAC	25mg to 75mg
Vitamin E	66mg (100iu) to 330mg (500iu)
Vitamin C	1,000 to 3,000mg
CoQ10	10mg to 50mg
Lipoic acid	10mg to 50mg
Anthocyanidin source	50mg to 250mg
or resveratrol	10mg to 20mg
Selenium	30mcg to 100mcg
Zinc	10mg to 20mg

There are several other supplements that really help boost your detoxification. MSM (methylsulphonylmethane) – a form of sulphur – is particularly helpful in supporting the liver. Aloe vera is also a great tonic for boosting the cleansing processes in the digestive tract (see page 165).

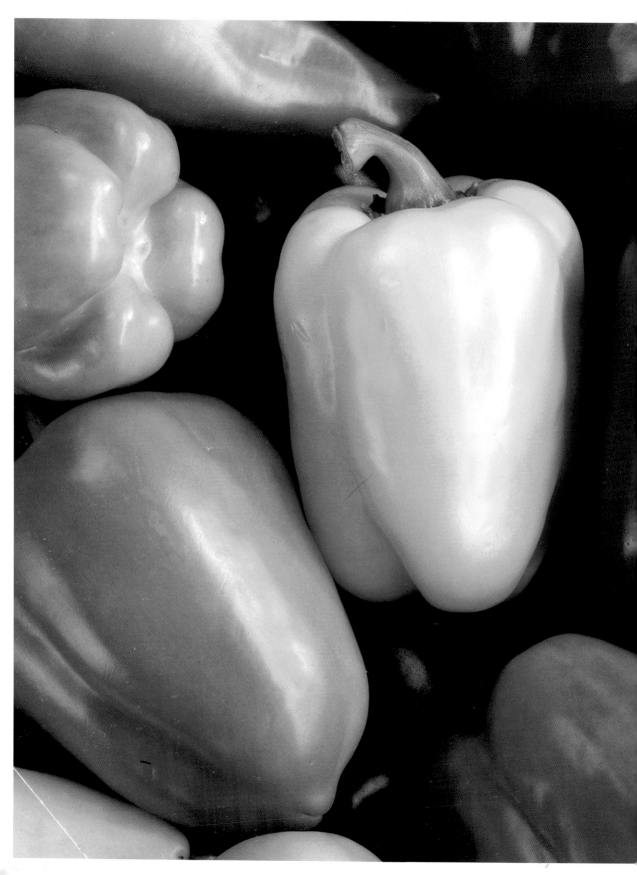

Nine-day detox plan

Throughout the centuries, health experts have extolled the value of spring-cleaning the body. In much the same way as you need time off sometimes to go on holiday, your body also benefits from a break from its work. This means stopping any foods or substances which increase your toxic load (i.e. alcohol, stimulants, refined foods) while increasing levels of all the nutrients which help your body heal and rejuvenate. Doing this once a year, for a week, can make a major difference to your energy levels.

- **Eat in abundance**
  Fruits – the most beneficial fruits, with the highest detox potential include fresh apricots, all types of berry, cantaloupe, citrus fruits, kiwi, papaya, peaches, mango, melons and red grapes
  Vegetables – especially good for detoxification are artichokes, peppers, beetroot, Brussels sprouts, broccoli, red cabbage, carrots, cauliflower, cucumber, kale, pumpkin, spinach, sweet potato, tomato, watercress and bean and seed sprouts

- **Eat in moderation**
  Grains – brown rice, corn, millet, quinoa: not more than twice a day
  Fish – salmon, mackerel, sardines, anchovies, trout: not more than once a day
  Oils – use extra-virgin olive oil for cooking and in place of butter, and cold-pressed seed oils for dressings
  Nuts and seeds – one handful a day of raw, unsalted nuts and seeds should be included: choose from almonds, Brazil nuts, hazelnuts, pecan nuts, pumpkin seeds, sunflower seeds, sesame seeds and flax seeds
  Potatoes and bananas – limit to one portion/one fruit every other day

- **Avoid**
  All wheat products – including bread, biscuits, cereals, pasta
  Meat, eggs and dairy produce (including milk, cheese, butter)
  Salt – and any foods containing it
  Bad fats – fried foods and anything containing hydrogenated fats
  Artificial additives – sweeteners, food additives and preservatives
  Dried fruit

- Begin your detox at the weekend or during a time when you don't have too much going on.

- Do some brisk exercise (i.e. walk or cycle) for at least 25 minutes every day, preferably in natural light.

- Drink at least 2 litres of water a day – purified, distilled, filtered or bottled. You can also drink herbal teas or dandelion coffee (which is good for the liver).

- Have half a pint of fruit or vegetable juice a day – either carrot and apple juice (you can buy these two separately and combine them with one-third water) with grated ginger, or fresh watermelon juice. The flesh of the watermelon is high in betacarotene and Vitamin C. The seeds are high in Vitamin E and antioxidant minerals zinc and selenium. You can make a great antioxidant cocktail by blending the flesh and seeds in a blender.

- Supplement two multivitamins/minerals, 2 grams of Vitamin C, two antioxidant complexes and 2 grams of MSM every day. Also have a shot of aloe vera juice.

Don't be surprised if you feel worse for a couple of days before you feel better. This is especially likely if you are eliminating foods to which you are allergic or upon which you are dependent.

Poor detoxification leads to inflammation

If you suffer with any inflammatory condition – asthma, arthritis, eczema, dermatitis or anything ending in 'itis' – your body is sounding an alarm bell. Basically, your toxic load has overpowered your system. Inflammation is usually accompanied by pain or irritation, so most people end up taking drugs, perhaps starting with painkillers or steroids, then moving on to antibiotics when infections set in. The drugs treat the symptoms but not the cause – in fact they usually aggravate the cause by irritating the gut and making the intestinal wall more leaky, which is what non-steroidal anti-inflammatory drugs and antibiotics do. This means that more garbage gets into the body, further overloading detoxification

The Drug Dilemma

Many medical drugs (such as painkillers or anti-inflammatory drugs) suppress the body's normal responses to an alarm signal. Instead of addressing the underlying problem, we take drugs to block the symptoms. They act like toxins in the body and can weaken the digestive and immune systems, which contribute to a further decline in health. As a result, you need another drug to counteract the symptoms! It's a downwards spiral.

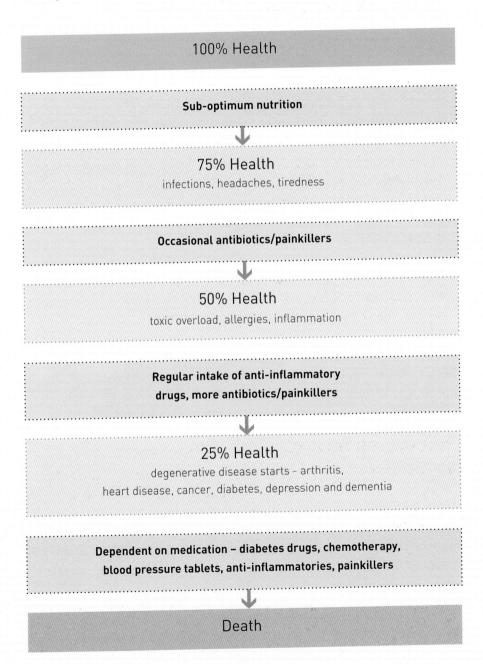

pathways (and also triggering food allergies – see page 63). Many drugs, such as paracetamol, are toxins in their own right and severely tax the liver. The result is ever-increasing overload on body systems, attracting more serious diseases and infections.

Drug-free painkillers

To avoid the damage caused by pharmaceutical drugs, consider natural anti-inflammatory alternatives.

- **Omega 3 fish oils** – these are converted in the body to anti-inflammatory substances. In trials, these have been shown to reduce inflammation from eczema, asthma and athritis. An effective amount is the equivalent of 1000mg of EPA, DPA and DHA a day, which means two or three capsules.

- **Turmeric** – this bright yellow spice contains the active compound curcumin, which has a variety of powerful anti-inflammatory actions. Trials in which it was given to arthritic patients have shown it to be similarly effective to the anti-inflammatory drugs, without the side effects. You need about 500mg, one to three times a day.

- **Boswellia** – derived from Frankincense, this plant is a very powerful natural anti-inflammatory agent that reduces joint swelling, restores and improves blood supply to inflamed joints, provides pain relief, increases mobility and prevents or slows the breakdown of cartilage. Preparations are available in tablet and cream form – the ideal dose is 200 to 400mg, one to three times a day; the creams are especially useful in the treatment of localised inflammation.

- **Ashwagandha** – this traditional Ayurvedic herb contains a powerful natural anti-inflammatory substance called withanolides that have been shown to be twice as effective as hydrocortisone. Try 1000mg a day of the root, providing 1.5 per cent withanolides.

- **IsoOxygene** – one of the most effective natural painkillers of all is this extract from hops. It works just as well as painkilling drugs but without the associated gut problems. You need about 1500mg a day.

- **Ginger** – as well as being anti-inflammatory, ginger is also rich in antioxidants. Supplement 500–2000mg a day in tablet form, or eat a 1cm slice of fresh ginger each day.

- **Polyphenols** – these antioxidant compounds are found in green tea, grape skins and onions and are particularly rich in olives (the active substance here is called hydroxytyrosol). Try 400mg a day.

- **MSM** – this stands for methylsulfonylmethane and is a source of the essential mineral sulphur. Sulphur is involved in a multitude of key body functions, including pain control, inflammation, detoxification and tissue building. Extraordinary results are starting to be reported in terms of pain relief and relief from arthritis, from supplementing around 3 grams of MSM daily.

It's possible to find many of these nutrients combined into single formulas. See the Supplement Directory (page 165).

Summary

You body is constantly working to make safe all the toxins that you encounter and create from everyday functions such as breathing and digestion. Supporting your liver – the main organ of detoxification – is essential to good health.

- Aim to reduce the toxic load on your body by reducing your consumption of alcohol, caffeine, refined carbohydrates and sugar.
- Also avoid recreational drugs, medicinal drugs (where possible), cigarettes and pollution and eat organic where possible.
- Filter your drinking water.
- Increase your intake of fresh fruits and vegetables and consider supplementing additional antioxidant nutrients.
- Once a year, do a week's detox programme to give your body a break.
- If you suffer with an inflammatory condition, address the underlying cause and consider natural anti-inflammatories rather than drugs.

FIND OUT MORE
Read *The Holford 9-Day Liver Detox*, by Patrick Holford and Fiona McDonald Joyce (published by Piatkus).

Increase Your Mood, Memory and Concentration

MOOD AND MEMORY QUIZ

☐ Is your memory deteriorating?

☐ Do you find it hard to concentrate and often get confused?

☐ Are you often depressed?

☐ Do you easily become anxious or wake up with a feeling of anxiety?

☐ Does stress leave you feeling exhausted?

☐ Do you often have mood swings and easily become angry or irritable?

☐ Are you lacking in motivation?

☐ Do you sometimes feel like you're going crazy?

☐ Do you suffer from insomnia?

☐ Do you have disperceptions where things don't look or sound right or you feel distant or disconnected?

☐ Does your mind ever go blank?

☐ Do you often find you can remember things from the past but forget what you did yesterday?

☐ Do you wake up in the early hours of the morning?

☐ Are you prone to premenstrual tension?

☐ Is your mood noticeably worse in the winter?

How do you score?

0-3 yes answers	4-6 yes answers	7 or more yes answers
You do not appear to be experiencing mood or memory problems – but that doesn't mean you won't in the future. Follow an optimum nutrition approach now to safeguard yourself.	You are beginning to show signs of reduced memory or declining mood. Identify your key areas and focus on improving these.	Your mind and mood are under pressure, so identify what's causing the stress and eliminate it, while increasing all the relevant nutrients.

Improving intelligence, memory and mood

Your IQ, mood and memory are not predetermined factors over which you have no control. Like the rest of your body, you can take steps to improve the health of your brain – so you can increase your IQ, enhance your mood and improve your memory.

Your brain and nervous system consists of an incredible network of special cells called neurons. Each neuron is capable of forming tens of thousands of connections with other neurons. This forms a huge web that represents all you know and feel. When you learn new things, you build new connections that actually change the wiring of your brain.

In the same way that hormones carry messages in the body, chemicals called neurotransmitters carry messages in the brain. For example, serotonin is the neurotransmitter that makes you feel happy.

Both your brain and neurotransmitters are made from nutrients. Therefore what you eat and drink has a big impact on how your brain functions and how you feel.

Hey, fat head!

Take out the water and your brain is made of 60 per cent fat. This is why essential fats are so important for mental function. The newspapers have been full of stories about how giving fish oils (which are rich in Omega 3 fats) to children helps to improve concentration and behaviour. Many scientific studies confirm that an optimal intake of these fats improves mood and intelligence at any age and also reduces aggression. Giving Omega 3 fats to people with depression, for example, can be more effective at lifting their mood than anti-depressant drugs.

Nutrients drive your brain

Neurotransmitters are made from protein, so ensuring you get enough in your diet is important for keeping you stable, happy and motivated. The functioning of your brain also depends on vitamins and minerals. Without them, you can't convert protein into neurotransmitters or fats into brain cells. An optimal intake of vitamins and minerals helps you to think faster and concentrate for longer. In one trial, instigated by ION nutritionist Gwillym Roberts, giving a vitamin and mineral supplement to school children increased their IQ score by seven points. And in elderly people, supplementing B vitamins can significantly improve memory.

Fish oils improve memory

Oily fish are rich in Omega 3 fats that benefit brain function, but they also contain another important family of brain nutrients – phospholipids. Probably the most important phospholipid is called phosphatidyl choline. This supplies the brain with nutrients to make a neurotransmitter called acetylcholine which is vital for memory. If you don't have enough, you may experience poor memory, lethargy, decreased dreaming and a dry mouth. Deficiency of acetylcholine is thought to be one of the major causes of senile dementia, which affects one in every seven people over the age of 75. Luckily, you can boost levels by taking choline with Vitamin B5, which enhances its action. Taken together, these nutrients have proved effective in enhancing memory and mental performance. The best supplemental source of phosphatidyl choline is lecithin. Lecithin also aids fat digestion. You can buy it as capsules or granules, which you sprinkle on food. However, not all lecithin is the same. Look at the label and make sure the product contains more than 30 per cent phosphatidyl choline. The recommended dose is 1 tablespoon a day.

The brain drain

While nutrients can improve mental function, anti-nutrients do the opposite. Caffeine is a prime example. Coffee, while commonly thought to improve concentration, actually diminishes it. A number of studies have shown that the ability to remember lists of words is made worse by caffeine. And a combination of caffeine and alcohol slows reaction time and, in one study, made subjects more drunk than alcohol alone. Caffeine is present in coffee, tea, chocolate, caffeinated and cola drinks.

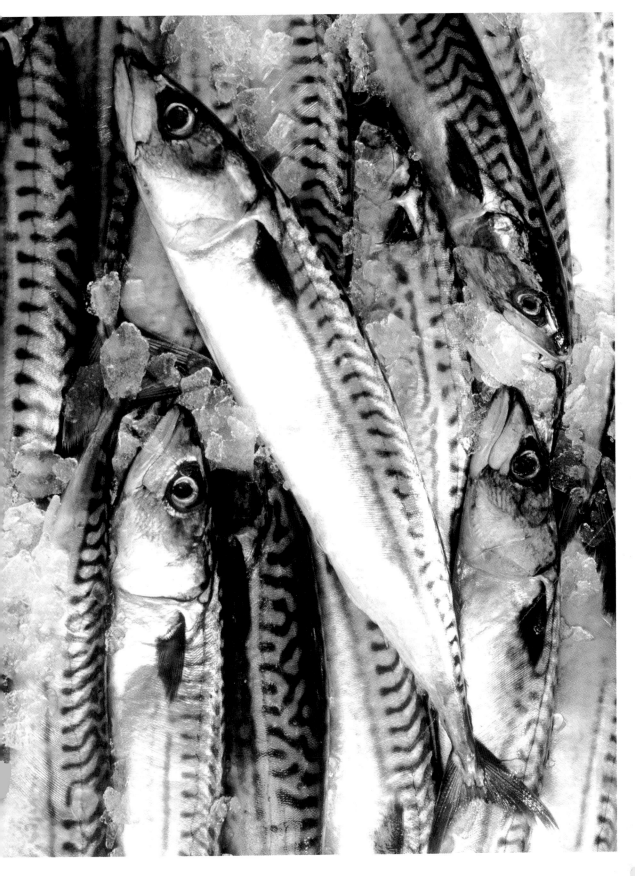

Nutrients Can Cure Depression

Depression can have a number of causes but many are finding amazing relief for this and other mental health problems by following an optimum nutrition approach. Doctors often prescribe anti-depressants, but these don't solve the underlying problem and more than half of those taking these drugs suffer with side effects. Amino acids (the building blocks of protein), essential fats and vitamins and minerals can provide the raw materials to bring the brain back into balance without any downside. For example, drugs such as Prozac help to increase levels of serotonin – the happy neurotransmitter. But in those taking Prozac, the suicide rate doubles. Taking a nutrient called 5-HTP, from which serotonin can be made, works better than anti-depressants without any dangerous side effects. It also helps reduce sugar cravings. Other studies prove the greater effectiveness of fish oils compared to anti-depressants.

If you suffer with low mood, try supplementing 100mg of 5-HTP* twice a day plus 1000mg to 2000g of Omega 3 fish oil and a good daily multivitamin and mineral. If you suffer with poor drive and motivation, instead of 5-HTP, try 500mg of tyrosine twice a day. This is an amino acid that increases levels of the motivating neurotransmitter dopamine. Also refer to my book *Optimum Nutrition for the Mind* to check out other possible factors – this covers issues such as toxicity, allergies, thyroid problems and biochemical imbalances that may also be a factor in depression and a range of other mental health problems.

A diet high in sugar and refined carbohydrates is another factor that reduces intelligence. Researchers at the Massachusetts Institute of Technology found that the higher the intake, the lower the IQ. In fact, the difference between the high sugar consumers and the low sugar consumers in the trial was a staggering 25 points! Sugar has also been implicated in aggressive behaviour, anxiety, hyperactivity and attention deficit, depression, eating disorders, fatigue, learning difficulties and premenstrual syndrome.

Toxic metals such as lead, mercury, cadmium and aluminium – which are present in our environment, in some drinking water, and in cigarette smoke – can accumulate in the brain and have been clearly demonstrated to affect mental health. Therefore keeping pollution to a minimum – which includes not smoking, drinking good quality, pure or filtered water and avoid using aluminium pans or foil – is a wise move for protecting your brain.

And finally, stress can play havoc with your brain function and affect your mood. If you are frequently stressed, take steps to reduce it and find ways to deal with it (see box on page 77).

Summary

Your brain function – which includes your IQ, mood and memory – relies on a good supply of the right nutrients to function effectively. Following an optimum nutrition diet will go a long way to supporting this. But if you want to improve your intelligence, memory or mood, also look to:

- Reduce your intake of stimulants such as coffee, tea, chocolate and cola, and of sugar and refined foods.
- Minimise your exposure to pollution and cigarettes.
- Make sure you are 'well oiled' with regular helpings of fish, seeds, their oils or essential fat supplements. You can also buy Omega-3-rich free-range eggs in supermarkets.
- Ensure that you achieve optimum nutrition through your diet and by taking a high-dose multivitamin and mineral supplement.
- Reduce stress and make some positive changes to your circumstances and the way you react to stressful situations.
- To improve memory, supplement an extra B complex containing 50mg of B5, plus take 1 tablespoon of lecithin granules (or capsules providing the equivalent) – choose a brand that contains more than 30 per cent phosphatidyl choline.
- To boost low mood, supplement 100mg of 5-HTP* twice a day plus 1000mg to 2000mg of Omega 3 fish oil.
- To boost poor drive and motivation, supplement 500mg of tyrosine twice a day.
* Don't take 5-HTP if you are already taking anti-depressant medication.

FIND OUT MORE
Read *Optimum Nutrition for the Mind*, by Patrick Holford (published by Piatkus).

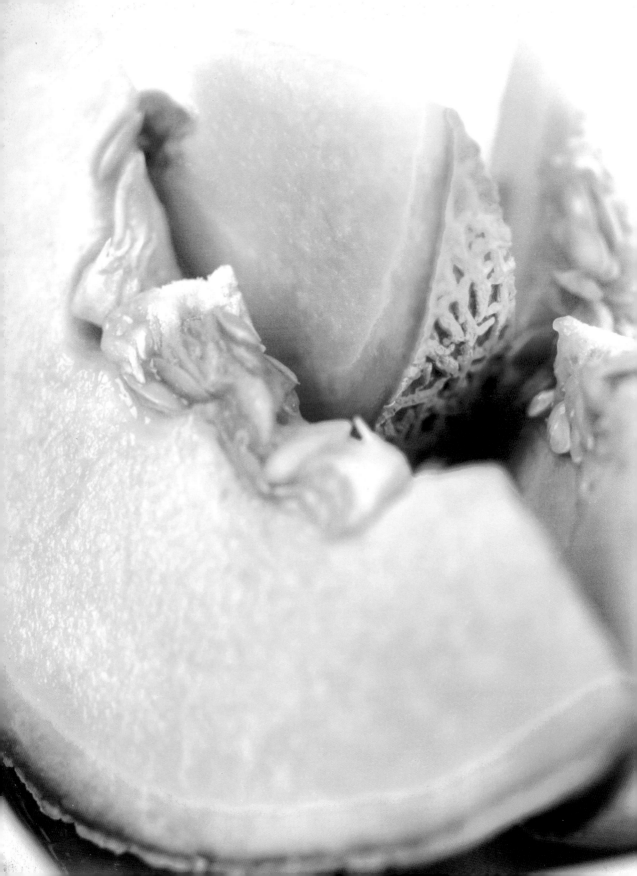

Part Three

Optimum Nutrition for Life

13. Good Food for Every Day

The rewards of eating a diet that optimises rather than depletes your health are many – more energy, great skin, sharper mind, better mood, trouble-free digestion, less illness... As you've seen in Parts One and Two, your food provides the raw materials from which you are made, so it makes sense to choose nutrient-rich varieties.

In Part One, you learnt about the best types of carbohydrate, protein and fat to eat. Chapter 7 introduced the concept of how to balance these food groups to ensure you have balanced blood sugar – which stabilises your energy and helps you achieve and maintain your ideal weight. Now we'll bring that all together to look at ideas for what to eat through the day – from when you get up to when you go to bed.

Fresh, whole foods – rather than processed, convenience foods – take a bit more effort to prepare than sticking a ready meal in the oven. However, you can still eat well simply and quickly, and without necessarily spending any more than you currently do on your weekly shop.

By following the low-GL principles for eating, which I explained in Chapter 7, you have an easy template for how to eat. This ensures you get a good balance of protein, slow-releasing carbohydrate and plenty of fresh vegetables and fruit (see plate illustration on page 102).

Some people prefer to follow specific recipes, so if the ideas here whet your appetite, I suggest you refer to one of the excellent cookbooks recommended (see page 107) for further inspiration.

Never skip breakfast

This is the most important meal of the day because, as its name suggests, you are 'break'ing the night 'fast'. Most people haven't eaten for 10–12 hours, so your body needs refuelling to ensure you start the day energised. If you're relying on fast-releasing carbohydrates (for example a slice of white toast and jam) or stimulants (a cup of coffee) to get you going, by mid morning your energy levels will be crashing. So start the day with a good source of slow-releasing carbohydrate and balance this with some protein. For example:

- A bowl of oat flakes (raw with milk or soya milk or cooked – you can add milk if you like, but oats are naturally quite creamy) with a cup of berries (look out for frozen packs in the supermarket) and maybe a small pot of live natural yoghurt (cow, goat, sheep or soya).

- A fruit power shake made by blending one tablespoon of mixed ground seeds (such as pumpkin, sunflower, sesame and flax seeds), 150g of live natural yoghurt or soya yoghurt, and a large handful of chopped fruit (e.g. plums, berries, apples, pears).

- A smoothie, using a tablespoon of my Get Up & Go shake powder (see Resources), with half a pint of milk (soya or rice), and berries or half a banana, plus a dessertspoon of ground seeds.

- A small serving of sugar-free muesli with a cup of milk (cow, goat, soya or rice milk).

- A bowl of fresh fruit salad with a handful of pumpkin/sunflower seeds and small pot of live natural yoghurt.

- Two thin slices of rye, granary or wholemeal toast or one thick slice, or three Nairn's rough oatcakes, with two eggs (boiled, poached or scrambled). Add some smoked salmon and plenty of black pepper. Or have a kipper with oatcakes.

- A two-egg omelette (plain or filled with whatever you fancy – such as mushrooms, watercress, cheese, cherry tomatoes, red onions, mixed peppers, fresh herbs). If you want a more portable option, pop the omelette into a wholemeal pitta bread to eat on the go.

- If you want toast and jam have nut butter (protein), such as almond butter with a sugar-free jam such as Meridian.

How to Balance What's on Your Plate

This provides a basic template to follow when you're preparing lunch or supper. Protein should make up a quarter of your meal; starchy carbohydrates (for example rice, potatoes, pasta or bread) another quarter; and half of your plate should be fresh low-carbohydrate vegetables or salad.

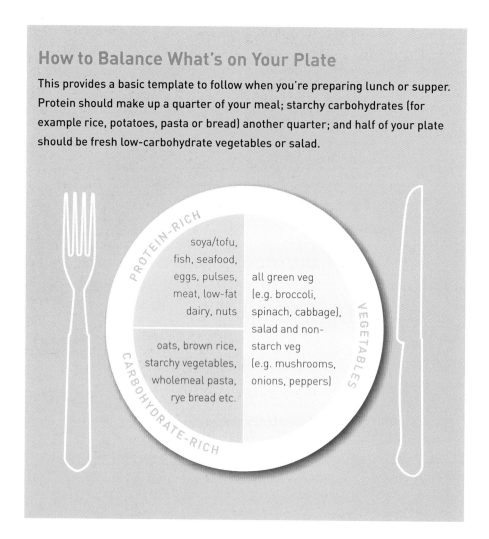

Protein options

For optimal health, the message is to eat more vegetable protein and fish, and less red meat and dairy. So experiment with new foods such as tofu – which you can buy marinated and ready to toss in to stir fries or salads. The protein-rich grain quinoa is easy to cook – just add 2 cups of water for every cup of quinoa, plus some vegetable stock and gently simmer for 15 minutes. Lentils, chickpeas and beans can be enjoyed in pâtés or dips (such as hummus) and can also be added to stews and pasta sauces for some high-fibre protein (buy ready to eat in tins, or soak your own from dried sources). And fish is easy to cook – steam, grill or bake with lemon and herbs. Tinned fish is also a cheap and easy way to add lean protein to a meal. For example, add some anchovies to a pasta sauce or mix wild salmon with cooked potatoes and onions to make a tasty fish cake (bind with an egg, season, dust with flour or cornmeal and grill).

Balancing carbohydrates

As you are probably beginning to realise by now, not all carbs are created equal. For optimal health, eat slow-releasing carbohydrates – i.e. those with the lowest GL score. Here are some examples of starchy (i.e. those that contain more sugar) carbohydrates with a glycemic load of seven (7GLs). That's what is recommended for people trying to lose weight on the Holford Low-GL Diet, as a main meal portion. If you just want to maintain your weight, you can increase the portion sizes suggested by about a third to 10GLs.

Starchy carb	7GLs looks like...	10GLs looks like...
Pumpkin/squash	large serving (186g)	double serving (266g)
Carrot	one large (158g)	two regular (266g)
Swede	regular serving (150g)	large serving (214g)
Quinoa	regular serving (120g)	large serving (188g)
Baked beans	large serving (150g)	double serving (214g)
Lentils	large serving (175g)	double serving (300g)
Kidney beans	large serving (150g)	double serving (214g)
Pearl barley	small serving (95g)	regular serving (136g)
Wholemeal pasta	half serving (85g)	large serving (112g)
White pasta	third serving (66g)	small serving (78g)
Brown rice	small serving (70g)	regular serving (84g)
White rice	third serving (46g)	half serving (66g)
Couscous	third serving (46g)	half serving (66g)
Sweetcorn	half a cob (60g)	one small cob (88g)
Boiled potato	two small (74g)	three small (106g)
Baked potato	one medium (59g)	one large (84g)
French fries	6–7 chips (47g)	8–10 chips (68g)
Sweet potato	half (61g)	one small (88g)

Non-starchy vegetables

You can enjoy these vegetables in unlimited quantities as their starch (i.e. sugar) content is minimal. Aim to fill half your plate with:

Alfalfa	Raw carrot	Kale	Rocket
Asparagus	Cauliflower	Lettuce	Runner beans
Aubergine	Celery	Mangetout	Spinach
Beansprouts	Courgette	Mushrooms	Spring onions
Raw beetroot	Cucumber	Onions	Tenderstem broccoli
Broccoli	Endive	Peas	Tomatoes
Brussels sprouts	Fennel	Peppers	Watercress
Cabbage	Garlic	Radish	

Ensure a regular intake of essential fats

As Chapter 2 explains, you have to get Omega 3 and Omega 6 essential fats from your diet. These fats support healthy mental function (e.g. concentration and mood), reduce inflammation in your body, keep skin soft, help balance your hormones and reduce your risk of developing killer conditions such as heart disease.

For Omega 3, the main source is oily fish – anchovies, sardines, herring, mackerel, salmon and trout. Eat three servings of these fish a week.

For Omega 6, the best dietary source are seeds – pumpkin, sunflower, flax seeds (also called linseeds), hemp and sesame – plus fresh, unsalted nuts such as walnuts, almonds, hazelnuts, Brazils and pecans. You can eat a small handful of nuts a day as a snack, or grind some seeds to sprinkle on cereal, yoghurt or salads. Grinding seeds helps to release their nutrients (otherwise you may swallow the smaller ones whole). You can grind them in a coffee grinder or food processor, then store them in a glass jar in the fridge to protect the delicate fats they contain. Even better, store your seed mix in the fridge, and grind fresh as you need them.

If you don't like fish or seeds, then it's vital to supplement essential fats on a daily basis to ensure you get a regular supply. I do both – eat seeds and fish and supplement daily essential fats. See page 166 for details of what to take.

Five Fast Food Ideas

Each of these meal suggestions can be cooked in 20 minutes or less. Balance quantities to fit the ideal plate ratios for protein, carbohydrate and vegetables.

- Salmon, chicken or turkey fillet coated in pesto and baked in the oven for 20 minutes, served with steamed cauliflower or broccoli, green beans and sweet potato.

- Cod baked for 20 minutes with cherry tomatoes, courgettes and red onion in olive oil and lemon juice, served with couscous and rocket or watercress.

- A packet of marinated tofu pieces, or strips of chicken, stir-fried with mixed vegetables (for example, onions, beansprouts, red pepper, cabbage), served with brown rice or noodles.

- Wholewheat or corn pasta tossed in tomato sauce (home-made or from a jar) with two handfuls of prawns or a tin of anchovies or tuna. Serve with a green salad or steamed spinach.

- Quinoa cooked in vegetable stock for 15 minutes and served with lightly steamed peas or mangetout and carrot, broccoli and red pepper (cut in strips) and a handful of lightly roasted cashew nuts.

Snacks for energy

Eating a snack mid morning and mid afternoon will help to maintain your energy levels through the day, so you don't get slumps or cravings for sweet foods or carbohydrates. To maintain stable blood sugar, stick to the slow-releasing carbohydrate with protein combination. For example:

- A piece of fruit, plus five almonds or a dessertspoon of pumpkin seeds

- A piece of bread or two oat cakes and half a small tub of cottage cheese (150g)

- A piece of bread/two oat cakes and half a small tub of hummus (150g)

- A piece of bread/two oat cakes and sugar-free peanut butter or another nut butter such as Meridian.

- Crudités (carrot, pepper, cucumber or celery sticks) and hummus

- Crudités and cottage cheese

- A small yoghurt (150g), no sugar, plus berries

- Cottage cheese plus berries

Healthy ways to prepare food

Cooking food for long periods or at a high temperature depletes nutrients. It also increases the rate at which the carbohydrate content will be released, because cooking starts to break it down (this is why an 8-minute steamed new potato has a lower GL score than an 70-minute oven baked potato). Having food raw, where appropriate, is the most nutritious way to eat it. But when you need to cook, the healthiest methods are steaming, boiling, poaching, steam-frying, baking and grilling – in that order. Avoid frying food as much as possible – and stay away from deep frying as if your life depended on it (because it does!).

Raw eating: Salad and fruit are not the only foods to enjoy raw. Raw vegetable sticks are a great way to start a meal, served with a dip, and raw vegetable juices provide a potent nutrient hit. You can even make raw soups like a Spanish gazpacho that are surprisingly delicious (blend together 225g ripe tomatoes, a clove of garlic, four spring onions, half a red pepper, 5cm length of cucumber – all chopped – with 225ml of passata, the juice of a lemon, 1½ tablespoons of olive oil, and salt and pepper).
Steaming: Instead of boiling your vegetables, steam them in a steamer, basket or even a colander over a pan of boiling water with a lid on top – this will preserve a lot more of their vitamins, as well as enhancing their flavour. You can also steam fish (especially the oily varieties, as this method doesn't damage the essential fats they contain).
Steam-frying: It's simple to do – just put a little oil into a pan that has a lid and sauté your food for a minute, creating enough heat. Then add a water-based sauce – such as a little vegetable stock, soya sauce, white wine or just some water – and put on the lid. The liquid prevents the oil getting too hot, and your food cooks fast but retains all its taste. This is a great way to cook stir-fries and vegetables.

Baking and grilling: This is a useful way of cooking fish or meat, but bear in mind that browning food creates harmful substances (oxidants), so avoid oil where possible and don't cook for too long.

Microwaving: Although quick, microwaving destroys more of the fat-based nutrients than steaming and can really damage essential fats, so avoid cooking oily fish this way. Microwaves also give off electromagnetic radiation which some researchers believe to be harmful.

And to drink?

Water is the most essential liquid to drink – aim to have the equivalent of six to eight glasses a day (which can include non-caffeine herbal teas or diluted juices). Other options include:

Coffee alternatives: All good health shops sell caffeine-free coffee substitutes such as Caro, Barley Cup or dandelion coffee. Teeccino is an American brand that's very close to real coffee – you brew it in a cafétière and it comes in a range of flavours, such as Original, Java, Mocha, Vanilla Nut.

Tea alternatives: If you're addicted to tea, try rooibos (red bush) tea with milk. Herb and fruit teas are also delicious, and widely available.

Fruit juices: Whether concentrated or fresh, fruit juices have a relatively high sugar content so ideally dilute half and half with water. The lowest in sugar is grapefruit juice, followed by apple then orange juice. Cherry juice concentrate (Cherry Active) is incredibly high in antioxidants and low GL. If you like fizzy drinks, dilute natural juices or cherry concentrate with fizzy water.

FIND OUT MORE
Read *Optimum Nutrition Cookbook* or the *Low GL Diet Cookbook*. Also great, especially if you have kids, is *Smart Foods for Smart Kids* (all published by Piatkus).

14. Superkids – Nourishing the Next Generation

What you feed your child to a large extent determines their health and dietary habits for life. As a parent, the time spent nourishing your child properly may be the greatest contribution you can make to their development.

Good health starts in the womb

Scientists are increasingly discovering that a mother's health and nutrition before conception and during pregnancy have a profound effect on the health of her child, and that patterns of disease in adulthood can be traced back to poor nutrition in the womb. A father's health is important too as poor diet and excess toxins can create defective sperm, which can account for up to 80 per cent of birth defects. For both would-be parents, optimum nutrition increases fertility (see page 80), the health of a pregnancy and the chances of having a healthy baby with strong resilience to disease.

The best odds for a healthy baby are achieved when both partners prepare for pregnancy. It takes three months for sperm and the egg or ovum to mature. If, during these pre-conceptual months, each partner pursues optimum nutrition, minimises his or her intake of anti-nutrients, especially alcohol, and stays well, the chances of a healthy conception are high.

Women who continue optimum nutrition once they've conceived also have a healthier pregnancy, which is good news for both mother and baby. Even the slightest deficiency can have serious effects on the health of a developing baby, and the idea that birth defects are often caused by nutritional imbalances in the mother is rapidly gaining wider acceptance. So far, slight deficiencies of Vitamins B1, B2 and B6, folic acid, zinc, iron, calcium and magnesium have all been linked to birth abnormalities. So too have excesses of toxic metals, especially lead, mercury, cadmium and copper (see page 38 for more on this). Eating a good diet, minimising toxins and supplementing beneficial nutrients are therefore essential for the healthy development of a baby.

Babyfoods – breast-feeding and weaning

Once a baby is born, the best way to continue to nourish him or her is by breast-feeding. Of course, a mother's milk is only as good as the raw materials her diet provides to make it, but the balance of nutrients in breast milk in an optimally nourished woman is far superior to those in formula milks. One key factor is the high levels of essential fats necessary for intellectual development – this is why children who were breast-fed have higher IQs. Other research has established that breast-fed babies are less prone to infections, digestive problems or allergies. And for the mother, breast-feeding not only helps to shift any excess pregnancy weight (it burns up an extra 500 calories a day), it also reduces her risk of developing breast cancer in later life.

The best gift you can give your child is to breast-feed them exclusively for six months. This is because their digestive tracts do not mature sufficiently before this time to tolerate any other type of food, and if they are exposed, then they are more likely to develop allergies. After six months, you can start to introduce your baby to the joys of solid food. When they stop sleeping through the night due to hunger – or start developing teeth – that's a good sign they are ready.

At the onset of weaning, give your baby food that is very easily digested – cooked, puréed vegetables and fruits are a good start (or choose sugar, salt- and additive-free organic pre-prepared baby purées). The longer you wait to give the most commonly allergenic foods, the less likelihood there is of your child developing an allergy to them. I recommend waiting until 9 months before introducing eggs or soya and 12 months for wheat, dairy, nuts and citrus. For all others, introducing one new food each day and being aware of any reaction (for example skin rash, eczema, runny nose, colic, diarrhoea, excessive sleepiness) will also help you to spot any other potentially allergenic foods. And like healthy adults, healthy babies need food that is fresh, organic, unprocessed, additive, salt and sugar free.

For as long as you continue to breast-feed in between solid feeds, you don't need to supplement your baby's diet with cow's milk. However, once you stop, you will need to ensure they get a good source of calcium. Despite popular belief, milk does not provide the best source of calcium – sesame seeds, sardines, almonds, spring greens, watercress, Brazil nuts and kale all provide more and are also high in other minerals, essential fats and protein (but I don't advise introducing nuts and seeds until your baby is a year old). At this point, adding ground seeds to cereals and soups, making dishes with lentils and beans, and including milk occasionally or calcium-enriched soya or rice milk is the best way to achieve an optimal calcium intake.

Develop good habits young

The taste for sugar is acquired through eating sweeter and sweeter foods. It can also be lost, usually with some resistance, by gradually reducing the level of sweetness in foods and drinks. This means replacing sweetened drinks with fruit juice, then gradually diluting them until you get half juice, half water. Of all the juices, grapefruit and apple contain the slowest releasing sugars, while grape juice contains the fastest releasing ones. Few children drink enough water. You can encourage your child to drink water by giving them a glass when they are thirsty, followed by a glass of diluted juice. Cherry concentrate diluted is excellent.

I don't advise giving sweets, sweetened foods, cola and other sweetened drinks as treats. If you do, these foods and drinks become associated with something good, and later in life your offspring may choose to treat themselves all the time. Instead give fresh fruit or orange or pineapple juice, diluted with fizzy water. Cola drinks are especially bad because most contain caffeine, an addictive drug. It is quite amazing, given that you have to be an adult to smoke and drink alcohol, that caffeine can be freely added to drinks advertised to children, who cannot read.

Very few breakfast cereals are truly sugar free. Food manufacturers help children to develop a sweet tooth at an early age: most processed cereals contain fast-releasing carbohydrates and have added sugar. Instead of giving your children such cereals, provide them with a choice of oats, sugar-free cornflakes or other such unsweetened wholegrain cereals, and encourage them to sweeten their cereal with fruit, such as a sliced banana, apple or pear, some berries or perhaps a few raisins.

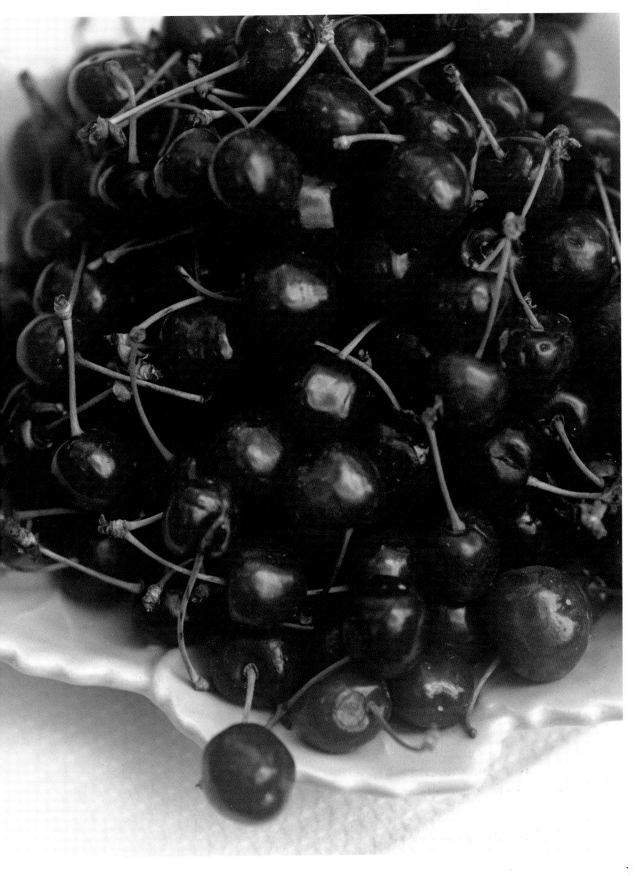

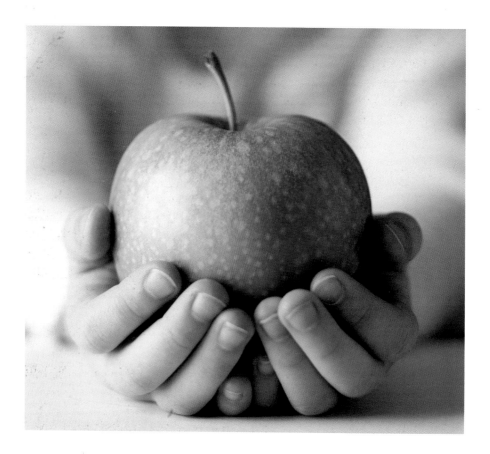

The best snack is fruit (especially berries), so make sure you always have a mountain of fresh, appealing fruit for your children to nibble on. Send them to school with fruit rather than money to buy sweets. Sure, when they are older and have pocket money they will buy sweets and get them at parties. But if sweets, sweetened drinks and sugary foods are not part of their day-to-day diet, they are unlikely to crave them or develop an addiction.

Another good habit to develop in your children is eating vegetables with each meal. The trick here is to find ways of preparing vegetables so that they taste good. Too many vegetables are cooked to death and taste bland. Raw organic carrots, peas, parsnip chips (made by slicing and baking on a tray with a drizzle of olive oil), and mashed and jacket-baked potatoes are naturally quite sweet and popular with children. Serving something raw with each meal, even if it is just a few leaves of watercress, grated red cabbage, tomato or carrot, develops the taste for salad foods.

While there are many ways of making healthy desserts, if a child always ends a meal this way they acquire a habit for life. Instead, restrict healthy desserts as a treat and give the child as much of the main course as he or she wants. If children are still hungry at the end of a meal, let them help themselves to fruit.

Who wants an 'average' child?

What is 'normal' behaviour in children? When we carried out the largest ever children's diet and behaviour survey – involving over 10,000 British school kids, aged between 6 and 16 years old – we found that more than one in three suffers from attention or concentration problems and mood swings or tantrums, with almost half having constant sugar cravings. Our Food for the Brain Child Survey (see Resources), also found that:

- The average intake of dark green vegetables is one serving a week.

- The average intake of seeds/nuts (high in essential fats) is half a serving a week.

- The average sugar serving in or added to food and drinks is 3.5 a day.

- Children who eat diets high in fried food or takeaways are three times more likely to be badly behaved.

- Children who eat vegetables, oily fish, nuts and seeds do best at school.

- Children with better diets have 11 per cent higher SAT scores.

When you understand that nutrients make the body work – and that our 21st-century junk-food diets are severely nutrient-depleted – these findings aren't that surprising. For example, the brain is 60 per cent fat. So children who eat good fats – from raw nuts, seeds and oily fish – double their chances of high academic performance. Children who eat damaged fats, in fried food and takeaways, are twice as badly behaved, as well as performing badly at school. In a sense these fats make your brain thicker and less responsive – and they appear to make children thicker too.

Improving attention problems

Many children with attention deficit hyperactivity disorder (ADHD) – which covers a whole range of behavioural problems – have known symptoms of essential fat deficiency such as excessive thirst, dry skin, eczema and asthma. Yet we know that supplementing essential fats can improve behaviour and learning in those with ADHD. Supplementing other nutrients vital for brain health – such as Vitamin A and zinc – can also have a dramatic impact on behaviour and performance in children. And the results can be seen very quickly.

In a trial for ITV's *This Morning* show, I devised a one-week experiment to put optimum nutrition to the test. From a class of 30 children aged six to seven years in a London primary school, the 12 who had learning, attention or behaviour difficulties were selected.

For one week the children and their parents were asked to not eat or drink foods containing added sugar or additives. The children were also asked to eat more fish and put seeds on their morning cereal (to increase essential fats). In addition, they were given a fruit juice drink with added vitamins.

In just one week, four out of the 12 children showed a dramatic improvement in behaviour, concentration, reading and writing. Reece was one of these children. He had real problems concentrating, sitting still, reading and writing at the beginning of the week. But by the end of the week, he had gone through a Jekyll and Hyde transformation: not only could he write one and a half pages, compared to only four lines before, but also his handwriting improved dramatically. His mother, who was sceptical about the project, said: 'I thought that nothing could calm this child down. We'd seen a psychologist but they didn't help. He was very fidgety, he was hard to get into bed, hyperactive and constantly on the go and with occasional tantrums. Now he's a completely different child. He's a lot calmer and he wants to do more at school. In two weeks his reading has gone up a level. He doesn't get so overexcited and he's much nicer to be with. We are definitely going to stick with the diet.'

Since then the Food for the Brain Foundation has run projects in primary schools, and schools for children with special educational needs, which has demonstrated significant improvements in learning and behaviour through applying optimum nutrition principles (see Resources for details and *www.foodforthebrain.org*).

Of course, not everything can be blamed on diet and nutritional deficiencies. As for adults, modern living is also proving stressful for children. Combine this with poor diet and too many children go over the edge into mental health problems. Some want to go further. Childline receives 1,500 calls each year from suicidal children. More than ever, our children need love, support and optimum nutrition.

Summary

Optimum nutrition is important at all stages of life, particularly prior to conception (for both women and men) and during pregnancy. Once your child is born, you can provide them with the best start in life by following the tips below:

- Breast-feeding is nutritionally far more beneficial than bottle feeding, as long as the mother is optimally nourished. So I recommend you eat a good diet (as outlined on page 43) and take a post-natal multivitamin and mineral supplement, together with an essential fat supplement.
- Do not wean your baby before six months, and then restrict the most common allergens (wheat, dairy, soya, citrus, nuts and eggs) until nine to 12 months.
- Once fully weaned, apply the same optimum nutrition diet principles to your child as to yourself.
- Restrict sweet foods and drinks to prevent your child from developing too sweet a tooth. Dilute fruit juices and give fruit for snacks instead of sweets.
- Encourage your child to eat vegetables with each meal, and serve some raw for added health benefits.
- Supplement your child's diet with a good multivitamin and mineral and essential fat supplement (see page 167 for details).
- Encourage your child to eat oily fish or nuts and seeds.

FIND OUT MORE
Read *Optimum Nutrition Before, During and After Pregnancy*; *Healthy Food for Healthy Kids* and *Smart Food, Smart Kids* (all published by Piatkus).

15. The Six Health Problems You Don't Have to Have

The vast majority of people die from preventable diseases. Obesity is the top preventable cause of premature death in the US. In the UK it's number two, just behind smoking. People are digging their own graves with their knife and fork.

The three diseases which cause the majority of deaths are cancer, heart disease and diabetes. All are associated with obesity. Every year in Europe, a million people are diagnosed with memory decline and dementia, many of who go on to develop Alzheimer's. And degenerative conditions such as arthritis and osteoporosis affect tens of millions in Britain. Yet all can be prevented and, in many cases, reversed, thus extending your healthy lifespan by ten or twenty years.

Osteoporosis: a silent epidemic

The epidemic of osteoporosis has made many women think seriously about the health of their bones. It is the silent thief that robs up to 25 per cent of your skeleton by the time you reach 50, without you even realising. Particularly prevalent in women after the menopause, it increases the risk of bone fractures that occur in one in three women and one in twelve men by the age of 70.

Supporting hormonal health naturally through and after the menopause is key for women (see Chapter 10). But diet also plays a big role in bone health – after all, in some cultures which don't eat a typical Western diet, there is no osteoporosis at all.

A key factor in our diet appears to be eating very high amounts of animal protein, such as meat two or three times a day, and insufficient sources of nutrient-rich plant foods (fruit and veg). Protein-rich foods are acid-forming. The body cannot tolerate substantial changes in acid levels in the blood so neutralises too much through two main alkaline agents – sodium and calcium. When the body's reserves of sodium are used up, calcium is taken from the bones. Therefore the more protein you eat, the more calcium you need.

To boost calcium intake, most people think 'milk'. Yet in some studies, women who drink more milk have a higher incidence of bone fractures than those who consume less. This is because, along with calcium, milk also contains protein – so it's acid-forming. Some scientists now believe that a lifelong consumption of a high-protein, acid-forming diet (from excess meat and dairy foods) may be a primary cause of osteoporosis.

Consuming less animal protein and more vegetable protein (for example grains, pulses, nuts and seeds) is associated with better bone health, as is boosting your intake of nutrients which support bone health. Calcium-rich foods include sesame seeds, tahini (sesame seed paste), kale, sardines, almonds, spring greens, watercress, Brazil nuts and kale – and all contain more calcium than milk. The other benefit of these foods is that they also contain other nutrients which are key to bone health. You see, along with calcium, phosphorus and magnesium are needed to build bone. Vitamin D is also important as without it, the body cannot absorb calcium. It is assisted by the mineral boron. Most of us don't get enough Vitamin D, which is made in the skin in the presence of sunlight. The best food source is fish. It's certainly worth supplementing extra. Vitamin C makes collagen (part of the bone structure), and zinc helps to make new bone cells. This orchestra of nutrients is often found in 'bone-friendly' supplements.

If you want to keep your bones in good health, pursue an optimum nutrition diet with these additions:

- Take regular weight-bearing exercise as this stimulates bone regeneration – so walk, run, dance or visit the gym three times a week. Also, climb the stairs rather than using the lift.

- Reduce your meat and dairy consumption and instead boost intake of vegetable protein sources (such as quinoa, pulses, nuts and seeds), as well as fish, and calcium-rich alternative milks.

- Reduce your stress level and keep stimulants to a minimum – both impact on bone health.

• Make sure your diet is rich in minerals from seeds, nuts, fresh fruit and vegetables.

• If you are post menopausal – or know your bone density is reducing – take a daily bone-supporting supplement (see the Resources section for details).

Combating arthritis, aches and pains

According to Dr Robert Bingham, a specialist in the treatment of arthritis, 'No person who is in good nutritional health develops rheumatoid or osteo-arthritis'. Yet by the age of 60, nine in every ten people have it. And this means living with pain and stiffness. The widespread belief is that there is nothing that can be done except to take painkillers, which more often than not speed up the progression of the disease (see page 89). But there are many proven ways to reduce pain and inflammation without drugs, even when degeneration is severe.

Fred is a case in point. He had seen many specialists and tried all the conventional treatments. Then he tried the optimum nutrition approach. 'I used to have constant pain in my knees and joints, could not play golf or walk more than ten minutes without resting my legs. Since following Patrick's advice, my discomfort has decreased 95–100 per cent. It is a different life when you can travel and play golf every day. I never would have believed my pain could be reduced by such a large degree, and not return no matter how much activity in a day or week.'

In addition to following an optimum nutrition diet, key strategies for reducing pain and inflammation are:

• Identify and avoid allergens (see page 64).

• Boost your intake of antioxidants via diet (see page 70) and in an all-round antioxidant supplement.

• Address high stress levels and keep stimulants to a minimum as both have a negative effect on joint health.

• If you have joint inflammation, take a daily supplement of 1000mg of EPA/DPA/DHA fish oil and a natural anti-inflammatory formula containing nutrients such as turmeric, boswellia or hop extracts, as well as glucosamine hydrochloride and MSM (see page 90 for more on natural anti-inflammatories).

FIND OUT MORE
Read *Say No To Arthritis* by Patrick Holford (published by Piatkus).

Sometimes aches and pains occur in the muscles and not the joints. This is not arthritis and may be due to one of two conditions.

The first is fibromyalgia, which is characterised by a number of tender points in specific muscles. This is believed to be due to a problem in the energy metabolism of the muscle cells, and not inflammation. A particular form of magnesium, magnesium malate, is proving very effective at relieving fibromyalgia – take 900mg of magnesium malate a day (3 capsules) providing about 100mg of magnesium and 800mg of malic acid, together with a supportive diet plus supplements. Stress, which uses up magnesium, makes this condition worse.

The second condition is polymyalgia, characterised by early morning stiffness, often in the shoulders and hips, and is often brought on when the body's detoxification systems are overloaded. It therefore usually responds to antioxidant supplementation and liver detoxification (follow the advice in Chapter 11). It's also worth checking your B vitamin status with a homocysteine test (see the box on page 123).

Say no to heart disease

You have a 33 per cent chance of dying from heart disease before you reach 75. That is the bad news. The good news is that heart disease is, in most cases, completely preventable.

Although the heart is the key organ in your cardiovascular system, the main diseases occur as a result of blockages in the arteries – the blood vessels which carry blood from your heart around your body. This is because the arteries get damaged and inflamed. When combined with thicker than normal blood containing clots, blockages can occur which stop the flow of blood. This is what causes angina, heart attack, most strokes or thrombosis.

High blood pressure also raises your risk of heart disease. It often occurs because, with age, blood vessels lose their elasticity and start to harden – making it harder for your heart to pump blood around the body.

A number of nutritional strategies have been shown to reduce high blood pressure and stop – even reverse – narrowing of the arteries. Reducing your intake of salt and increasing sources of magnesium, calcium and potassium can make a substantial difference to blood pressure in just a month. It's well worth supplementing an extra 300mg of magnesium, as well as eating more greens and pumpkin seeds, which are excellent food sources. Omega 3 fats (in oily fish and fish oil supplements) thin the blood, reduce inflammation and lower your risk of heart disease. Antioxidants also protect arteries. Supplementing a combination of these nutrients is more effective in the long term than taking drugs designed to lower blood pressure, as the nutrients deal with the cause of the problem, rather than the symptom.

Keeping cholesterol in check

Cholesterol has become a dirty word, and while it's true too much increases your risk of arterial disease, not having enough is also bad news for health. It's needed by your body to make hormones and for healthy brain function.

Blood tests report two kinds of cholesterol – LDL and HDL. The HLD (short for high-density lipoprotein) variety is better because it carries cholesterol away from your arteries. Having a higher HDL cholesterol reduces your risk of heart disease, while having a higher LDL increases your risk. Ideally you want half to one third of your total cholesterol as HDL.

Once again, a low GL diet, plus optimum nutrition supplements are highly effective at achieving the ideal cholesterol balance. Extra Vitamin B3 (niacin) will lower cholesterol and increase healthy HDL levels, although you need to supplement 500–1,000mg a day. The same is true for Omega 3 fish oils. These measures are at least as effective – and in most cases more so – than cholesterol-lowering statin drugs and, of course, have none of the side effects of statins.

Supernutrition for a healthy heart

The following guidelines apply to us all as a means of eliminating risk and adding at least ten healthy years to our lifespan:

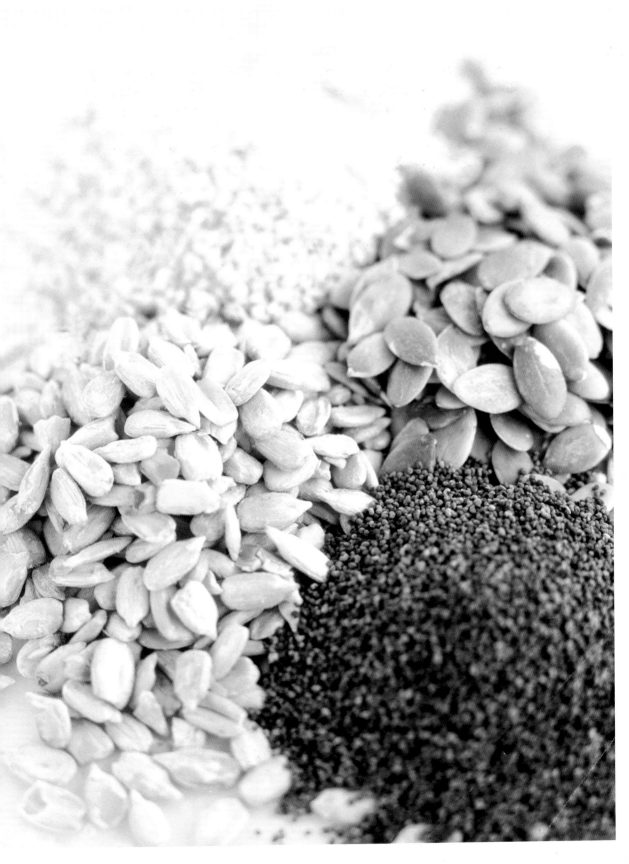

Ideal Test Scores for Cardiovascular Health

	High Risk	Medium Risk	Healthy
Cholesterol (UK)	‹ 3.1 or › 8.5mmol/l	› 6.2mmol/l	4–5.2mmol/l
Cholesterol (US)	‹ 120 or › 330mg/dl	› 240mg/dl	150–200mg/dl
Total Cholesterol/HDL	› 8:1	› 5:1	‹ 3.5:1
Blood Pressure	› 140/90	› 130/85	‹ 125/76
Pulse	› 85	‹ 85	‹ 70

› = more than   ‹ = less than

- Avoid fried food and limit your intake of meat and foods high in saturated fat. Oily fish such as mackerel, salmon and sardines are better.

- Eat plenty of fresh fruit and vegetables, which are high in calcium, magnesium and potassium, especially green leafy vegetables and beans, which are high in folic acid.

- Eat oats and rough oat cakes, such as Nairns, high in beta-glucans, a cholesterol-lowering soluble fibre high in oat bran.

- Do not add salt when cooking, or to your plate, and restrict your consumption of foods with added salt.

- Keep fit, not fat.

- Don't smoke.

- Avoid prolonged stress.

- Know your blood pressure and have your blood lipid level checked every five years.

B Vitamins Can Reduce Risk of Death

We all have a substance in our blood called homocysteine. It's produced when the liver breaks down protein from our food and should ideally be converted into other substances which are beneficial for our health. However, like any process in the body, this conversion relies on enzymes – and these enzymes are powered by B vitamins, which are often lacking in the modern diet. The result is that homocysteine levels rise – and with them, your risk of developing diseases, particularly heart disease. Research has found that having a high level of homocysteine in your blood is as great a risk factor for developing cardiovascular disease as having high cholesterol, and a much better indicator of stroke risk.

High homocysteine is also a risk factor for depression and memory decline, especially Alzheimer's, and many other diseases. But the good news is that it's easy to reduce high levels – and doing so will reduce your risk of death from any condition. You just need to have a simple blood test (there's even a home test that only requires a pin-prick blood sample – see Resources), then take a combination of nutrients to reduce your level. These include folic acid, B12 and B6. The ideal amount to supplement depends on your homocysteine level (see *www.thehfactor.com*), but suffice it to say that anyone should be supplementing at least 200mcg of folic acid, 12mcg of Vitamin B12 and 20mg of B6.

- Take an all-round antioxidant supplement including at least 400mg of Vitamin E, plus co-enzyme Q10, glutathione, alpha-lipoic acid and resveratrol, and 2 grams of Vitamin C, plus the Omega 3 fats EPA and DHA and a multivitamin containing B6, B12 and folic acid.

If you have cardiovascular disease or high blood pressure, the following also apply:

- See a nutritional therapist and have your blood lipid levels and homocysteine (see box above) measured.

- If you have high cholesterol and low HDL, take 1 gram of niacin a day. Niacin, in high doses, makes you blush. However, non-blushing forms of niacin are available in health food stores and on prescription.

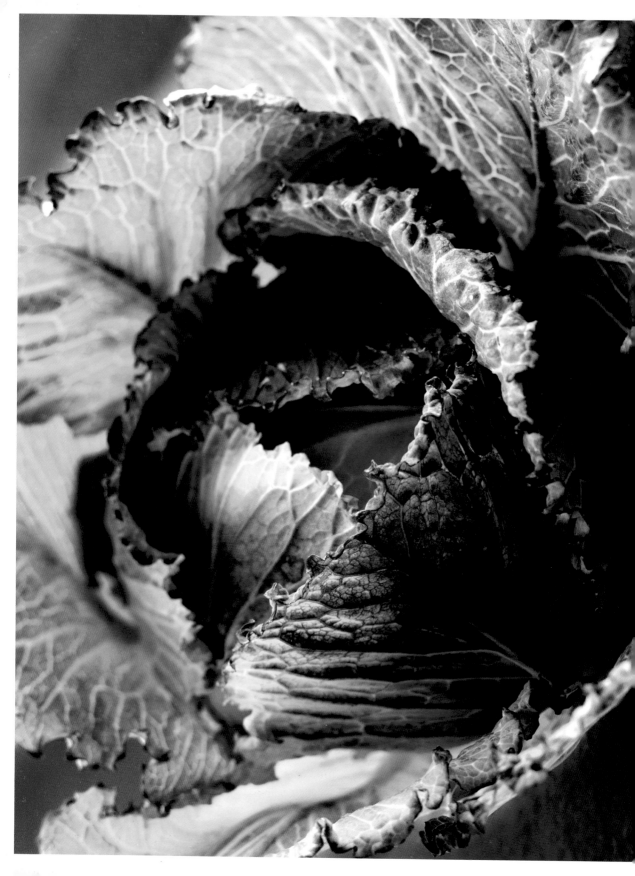

- If you have high cholesterol or triglycerides, take an EPA fish oil supplement giving you 1000mg of EPA.

- If you have high homocysteine, increase your intake of Vitamins B6, B12 and folic acid and other homocysteine modulating nutrients (see *www.thehfactor. com* for amounts).

- If you have high blood pressure, take 150mg of magnesium twice a day, in addition to 150mg in your multivitamin (450mg in total).

- Do all you can to improve your diet and lifestyle.

FIND OUT MORE

Read *The H Factor* by Patrick Holford and Dr James Braly (published by Piatkus).

Avoid diabetes

Type II or adult-onset diabetes is highly preventable, yet more and more young people are developing it. The obesity 'epidemic' in the West has helped fuel this rise. If you are obese, the risk of developing diabetes goes up 77 times! By 2010, one in six people over 40 is expected to have diabetes.

Diabetes is an extreme form of blood sugar imbalance. After years of struggling with blood sugar highs and lows – which we looked at in more detail in Chapter 7 – the body is unable to produce sufficient insulin (the hormone that helps to carry glucose out of the blood and into cells to make energy), or becomes insensitive to it. The result is too much glucose in the blood and not enough for the cells. Weight gain and fatigue are common in diabetics – as is increased risk of cardiovascular disease and eye and nervous system degeneration, because too much sugar in the blood damages arteries and tissues.

The early warning signs are similar to those of mild glucose imbalance (see the quiz on page 52), but they rarely go away as a result of simple dietary changes. One of the tell-tale signs is a continuous raging thirst as the body tries to dilute the excess blood sugar by stimulating us to drink. Of course, if you drink sugary drinks you make matters worse.

Getting blood sugar balanced again

The key to avoiding diabetes – or managing and even reversing it once you have it – is to keep your blood sugar level even. This is achieved best by eating little and often, choosing foods that contain slow-releasing carbohydrates and eating them with protein – following the basic tenets of a low GL diet explained in Chapter 7. Also important is avoiding all sugar and forms of concentrated sweetness, such as fruit juice and high-sugar fruits like dates, bananas and dried fruit. And cut out stimulants such as tea, coffee, alcohol and cigarettes.

FIND OUT MORE
Read *The Holford Low-GL Diet* by Patrick Holford (published by Piatkus).

In terms of supplements, the mineral chromium can help make the body more receptive to the insulin you are able to produce, which will encourage more sugar to be removed from the blood and converted to energy in the cells. Aim to have 200mcg a day, although diabetics respond best to 500 to 600mcg a day. Cinnamon also helps stabilise blood sugar, so the combination of chromium plus cinnamon is particularly effective.

Exercise is also helpful at reversing adult-onset diabetes – even a short walk after a main meal can reduce high blood sugar.

Conquering cancer

Cancer is the second greatest cause of death in the Western world. In the UK, one in three people are diagnosed with cancer during their lives and one in four currently die from it.

Cancer occurs when cells start to behave differently, growing, multiplying and spreading. It is like a revolution in the body, where a group of cells stop working for the good of the whole and run riot. The odd revolutionary cell is a common occurrence and the body's immune system isolates and destroys such offenders. However, in cancer, the immune system is overcome and the damage spreads.

Most cancers are primarily the result of changes that humans have made to our environment – what we eat, drink and breathe. According to one of Britain's top medical scientists, Sir Richard Doll, 90 per cent of all cancers are caused by such environmental factors. Even the most conservative experts say that at least two-thirds of cancers are associated with environmental and lifestyle factors.

Conventional treatments see cancer as the enemy and cut it out, burn it out through radiation or drug it out with chemotherapy. All these treatments weaken the body and don't address the underlying causes. Nutritional approaches to cancer aim to strengthen the body's immune system, remove potential cancer-causing agents and increase antioxidant nutrients which can fight the cancer naturally.

Hormone-related cancers

Many cancers of the breast and ovaries in women, and of the prostate and testes in men, appear to be related to an excess of hormonal 'growth' signals. We now know, for example, that oestrogen and synthetic progestin given in HRT increases risk of breast cancer.

Other factors that can cause hormone imbalances are prolonged stress and exposure to environmental chemicals from pesticides and industrial pollution (as discussed in Chapter 11). A high intake of dairy products also increases risk of hormonal cancers. Countries that have low or no consumption of dairy produce have remarkably low incidences of both breast and prostate cancers, as well as other hormone-related cancers. For example, the incidence of breast cancer in rural China is 1 in 9,000 women, compared to our incidence of 1 in 9, and prostate cancer, which affects 1 in 7 men in Britain, is virtually unheard of. In case you are wondering whether there's something inherently different in Asian people, their risk goes up when they immigrate to the US or UK. The main reason for the link between milk and these cancers, as well as colorectal cancer, is due to a hormone called Insulin-like Growth Factor (IGF-1) that milk elevates. This specifically promotes the growth of pre-existing cancer cells.

To reduce your risk of these types of cancer, consider alternatives to HRT (see page 79), deal with stress (see page 77), up your intake of antioxidants, reduce your exposure to environmental toxins by following the advice in Chapter 4, reduce your intake of dairy products, alcohol and fried fatty foods and lose weight if you need to. These measures are part of following an optimum nutrition approach, so you need do nothing extra than following the general advice in this book.

Cancer-fighting foods

Eating certain kinds of foods is associated with a decreased risk of cancer.

- Fruit and vegetables are top of the anti-cancer foods. These are good sources of Vitamins A and C and research links a high intake with reduced risk of cancer.

- Garlic, used liberally, is thought to help prevent cancer, probably because it contains sulphur compounds which help deal with toxins and free radicals.

FIND OUT MORE
Read *Say No to Cancer* by Patrick Holford (published by Piatkus).

- Soya beans, and beans and lentils in general, are associated with a lower risk of breast and prostate cancer. In Japan and China, for example, where soya is eaten as tofu, tempeh and miso, breast-cancer rates are hundreds of times lower than in the West.

- Live yoghurt may protect against colon cancer, as it contains bacteria that have been found to slow down the development of colon tumours. However, dairy-free probiotic supplements may be wiser.

- Sesame and sunflower seeds are rich in selenium, Vitamin E, calcium and zinc. Eating a spoonful every day will keep your antioxidant army in top condition.

Preventing dementia and Alzheimer's

Every day, four double-decker buses full of people are diagnosed with dementia. Three-quarters of these will go on to develop Alzheimer's disease, a condition that already clocks up more healthcare costs than cancer and heart disease. It is very likely that age-related memory decline and Alzheimer's disease are primarily caused by insufficient B vitamin intake (B vitamins are needed to keep homocysteine low – see box page 123) and excess oxidation and inflammation, again directly influenced by diet. This is good news because it means that Alzheimer's disease should be preventable and age-related memory decline reversible, at least in the early stages.

Alzheimer's disease and dementia have similar causes and associated risk factors to other common degenerative diseases, including cardiovascular disease and diabetes, both of which are largely preventable by optimum nutrition. The following measures can help you reduce risk factors:

- Follow an optimum nutrition diet (see Chapter 5).

- Increase your intake of the anti-inflammatory essential Omega 3 fats EPA, DPA and DHA (by eating oily fish and also taking a supplement).

- Increase your intake of the protective antioxidants such as Vitamins E and C (see pages 157 and 158 for food sources), as well as glutathione (in onions and garlic), anthocyanidins (in berries) and resveratrol (in red grapes and wine).

- Address high or prolonged stress to reduce high levels of the stress hormones, which can damage the brain.

- Test and reduce high levels of a harmful substance in the blood called homocysteine (see box on page 123). This is most important and requires amounts of B vitamins such as B6, B12 and folic acid at levels much higher than the RDA, plus other nutrients such as Trimethylglycine (TMG). Some supplements, designed to support healthy homocysteine levels, contain all of these.

FIND OUT MORE
Read *The Alzheimer's Prevention Plan* or *New Optimum Nutrition for the Mind*, both by Patrick Holford (published by Piatkus).

- Exercise your brain every day – learn something new, do a crossword or play a number game.

Once brain-cell degeneration occurs, levels of the brain's memory molecule – a substance called acetylcholine – start to decline. There is also growing evidence that nutrients that support acetylcholine production can help to improve cognitive function. The main players that have been shown to have some positive effect are called phosphatidyl choline, phosphatidyl serine and DMAE. These are all available as supplements (see the Supplement Directory for details). Eggs are especially rich in phosphatidyl choline.

16. Stay Young and Beautiful

Slowing the ageing process

The quest for never-ending youth and immortality is nothing new. Since the beginning of history, myths and legends abound about magic potions and people living for hundreds of years. And while this may be the stuff of fantasy, modern science can now provide some genuine understanding of how we can realistically extend our lifespan and prevent the problems of getting older. It's important to achieve both – after all, who wants to live to 100 if it means spending the last few decades of your life physically malfunctioning, in pain and losing your marbles?

In the last chapter, we explored how improving your diet and intake of beneficial nutrients can reduce your risk of the most common degenerative diseases – from arthritis to heart disease and Alzheimer's to cancer.

When it comes to slowing down the ageing process – so you stay looking and feeling younger for longer – the best results in research studies have consistently been achieved by giving animals low-calorie diets high in antioxidants and other nutrients. In other words, eating enough to maintain an ideal weight (so reducing fatty or sugary foods) and getting plenty of beneficial nutrients at optimum levels.

This reduces what's called 'oxidative stress' – the mechanism that causes you to age, where processes in the body and exposure to toxins and pollution create rogue molecules called free radicals that 'oxidise', or damage, your cells.

Although long-term human trials are still to be completed, there is every reason to assume that the same principles apply to us. Already, studies show that the risk of death is substantially reduced in those with a high intake of antioxidants. And anti-ageing expert Professor Denham Harman, from the University of Nebraska Medical School, believes the 'chances are 99 per cent that free radicals are the basis for ageing'.

Testing Your Antioxidant Potential

Your ability to stay youthful and healthy depends on the balance between your intake of harmful free radicals and your intake of protective antioxidants. As the scales start to tip away from health, early warning signs start to develop, like frequent infections, difficulty shifting an infection, easy bruising, slow healing, thinner skin or excessive wrinkles for your age.

Another sign of impaired antioxidant status is a reduced ability to detoxify the body after an onslaught of free radicals. So, for example, if you feel groggy or achy after a burst of exercise or after exposure to pollution (such as being stuck in a traffic jam or a room full of cigarette smoke), your antioxidant potential may need a boost.

There are also tests you can do via a nutritional therapist to measure your blood levels of antioxidant nutrients. See the Resources section for details of how to find one in your area.

This means that the key to longevity lies in reducing our exposure to free radicals (harmful molecules) and increasing the body's protection against them by increasing our intake of antioxidants. Reducing your exposure to toxins and increasing your intake of beneficial nutrients is one of the key principles of optimum nutrition, so if you follow the advice in this book, then you will already be on your way to achieving this.

Also important are homocysteine-lowering B vitamins because they improve a process in your body called 'methylation' and this enables you to better repair damaged DNA, which slows down the ageing process.

The best antioxidant nutrients

While the roles of antioxidant Vitamins A, C and E are well known, there are other important nutrients that also slow down the ageing process. Two of these are alpha-lipoic acid and carnitine. Studies involving feeding these to old rats have shown amazing reversals of ageing. Professor Bruce Ames, a molecular biologist at the University of California, who led this research, said of the supplemented animals: 'The brain looks better, they are full of energy – everything we looked at looks like a younger animal. It's the equivalent of making a seventy-five to eighty-year-old person act middle-aged.'

But can we apply all this to humans? To date, the circumstantial evidence is remarkably consistent across a wide variety of species and there is no reason to believe that human beings will be any different. And while you can eat sources of the main antioxidant nutrients, the only way to boost alpha-lipoic acid and carnitine is to supplement them.

Antioxidants: the Best Foods

Every year, more and more antioxidants are found in nature, including substances in berries, grapes, tomatoes, mustard and broccoli, and in herbs such as turmeric and ginkgo biloba. There are also thousands of beneficial substances in plant foods which are called phytonutrients, as we discussed on page 24. At the Institute for Optimum Nutrition, we did some research into the best fruits and vegetables, assessing the top five for each, based on a number of anti-ageing criteria. This included looking at their 'ORAC' rating, which measures antioxidant potential, and also at how much Vitamin C, folic acid, zinc and a potent anti-ageing phytonutrient called glucosinolate they contain. Here are the results:

	Zinc	Folic Acid	ORAC	Gluco-sinolate	Vitamin C	Total
TOP 5 VEG						
Tenderstem broccoli	5	3	4	5	4	21
Curly Kale	3	4	5	3	5	20
Spinach	5	5	4	3	2	19
Asparagus	4	5	2	3	1	15
Broccoli	3	3	2	3	3	14
TOP 5 FRUIT						
Strawberries	5	3	4	4	5	21
Blueberries	4	5	5	5	2	21
Raspberries	3	3	4	4	5	19
Oranges	3	4	3	3	5	18
Red Grapes	5	5	2	2	2	16

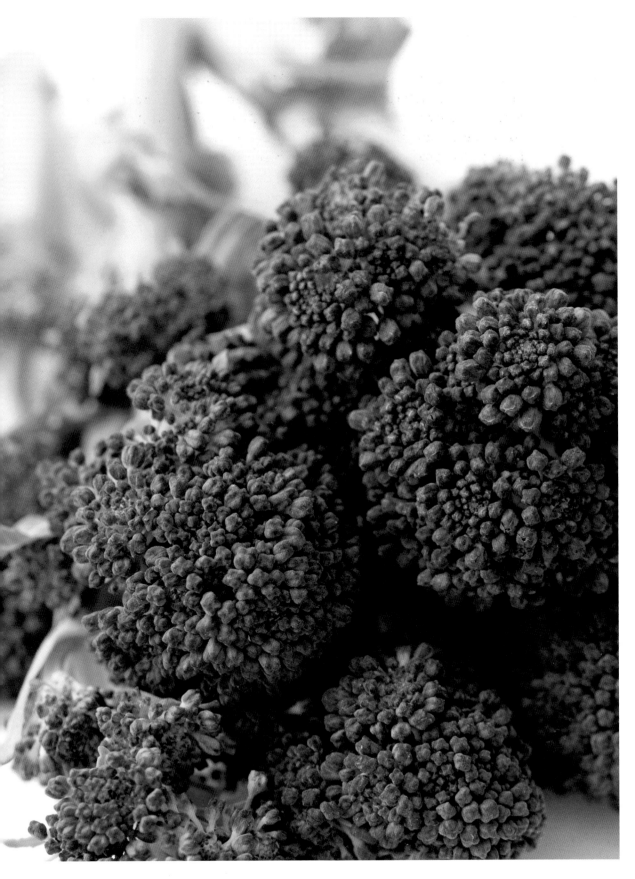

Feed Your Skin

One of the key signs of ageing is the condition of your skin. Every adult wants to look younger than their years – and having smooth, clear skin helps you achieve this.

Nutrition is fundamentally involved at every stage of skin development. Vitamin C is essential to make collagen (the fibre in the inner layer that keeps skin smooth and plump); essential fats keep skin cells soft and supple; Vitamin A replenishes skin and impedes the development of wrinkles; zinc aids new skin cell production and keeps skin elastic – a deficiency can result in stretch marks; and antioxidant nutrients such as Vitamins A, C and E and selenium protect against damage from sun and pollution.

Your skin is a remarkable barometer of your body's health and as such, is very much affected by how well you are internally. So getting all your body systems working optimally is crucial to addressing skin problems. Acne, for example, can be the result of a hormone imbalance – sometimes too much dairy; eczema can be due to food intolerances or impaired detoxification; and dry skin is a common sign of deficiency of essential fats and water in the diet.

Many common nutritional factors are involved in a wide variety of skin problems. To achieve healthy skin, follow the guidelines for reducing ageing and incorporate the following:

- Limit alcohol, caffeine, chemical additives, salt, saturated fat, sugar and smoking.

- Ensure a good supply of essential fats from oily fish (three times a week) and fresh nuts and seeds or cold-pressed seed oil (daily).

- If you are prone to dry skin or skin inflammation, supplement both Omega 3 and borage oil or evening primrose oil containing 200mg of the active Omega 6 fat, GLA, each day.

- Use a cream containing significant amounts of Vitamins A and C in forms that can penetrate the epidermis (such as ascorbyl palmitate or, even better, tetraisopalmitate, retinol or retinyl acetate or palmitate). This is proven to prevent wrinkles. See Resources, page 163.

- Limit exposure to strong sunlight and apply a sun-protection factor to your skin.

- Wash your skin with water, or a gentle oil-based cleanser, rather than soap.

FIND OUT MORE
Read *Solve Your Skin Problems*, by Patrick Holford and Natalie Savona (published by Piatkus).

Exercise keeps you young

Regular exercise can add seven years to your lifespan, conclude Dr Rose and Dr Cohen of the Veterans' Administration Hospital in Boston. But the exercise must be continued late into life and must be aerobic – that is, your heart rate must reach 80 per cent of its maximum for at least twenty minutes. Cycling, swimming and running are good; weightlifting and strengthening exercises, on the other hand, do little to extend your life (though they do have other benefits). Aerobic exercise reduces blood cholesterol levels, pulse rate and blood pressure, promoting better cardiovascular health as well as increasing mental function. It also helps you to maintain proper blood sugar control and is therefore especially helpful for diabetics.

Summary

It's possible to slow down the rate at which you age and enjoy a longer, healthier lifespan if you follow optimum nutrition principles. Specifically:

- Stay away from avoidable sources of free radicals – fried or browned food, exhaust fumes, smoke and strong sunlight.
- Eat plenty of antioxidant-rich fruit and vegetables (aim for at least five, and preferably seven to eight, portions each day).
- Don't eat processed, refined or sugary foods.
- Drink 1.5–2 litres of water each day, either plain or in herbal teas or diluted juices and drink alcohol infrequently – ideally red wine.
- Eat what you need to stay fit and healthy – but no more.
- Keep fit with a moderate (not excessive) amount of aerobic exercise.
- Manage your stress levels – reduce if necessary – and take time out each day to relax.
- Get seven hours of quality sleep each night.
- Take extra antioxidant nutrients – including Vitamins A, C and E, selenium and zinc, plus glutathione, alpha-lipoic acid, co-enzyme Q10 and carnitine. Ideally take an all-round antioxidant supplement in addition to an optimum nutrition multivitamin and extra Vitamin C.

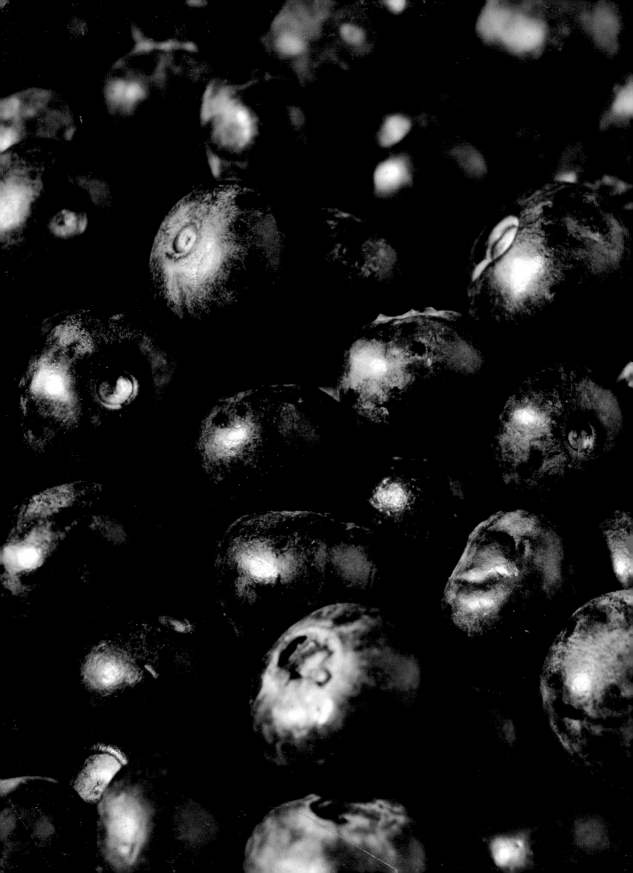

Part Four

Your Action Plan

17. Putting All You've Learnt into Practice

Congratulations – you've reached the part where you can start planning how you're going to put all you've learnt into action!

By now, I hope you are getting the hang of what optimum nutrition means. In Part One, we covered the basics of diet and supplements. If you've worked your way through the questionnaires in Part Two, you'll also have identified specific areas where your health could benefit from some attention. Now, we can bring it all together to help you formulate your personal 100% Health Action Plan.

Be bold and realistic

You will get the best results by really going for it. That means really improving your diet as best you can and taking the right supplements for a month. I encourage you to make a decision to change your habits for these four weeks. This takes discipline. The results are worth it.

At the same time, don't set yourself up for failure. Set yourself achievable goals. For example, if you currently drink five coffees every day, quitting all in one go might be pushing it. However, allowing yourself two a day for the first week, then one in the second week, then quitting in week three might be more achievable. So, set your ideal goals, then ask yourself 'is this achievable and realistic?' Here are the best diet goals to shoot for.

Diet goals

As we explored in Part One, there are ten basic diet goals to aim for:

1. Eat one handful of fresh seeds or nuts (whole or ground) – or one tablespoon of a cold-pressed seed oil a day.

2. Eat two servings of beans, lentils, quinoa, tofu (soya), 'seed' vegetables or other vegetable protein – or one small serving of lean meat, fish, cheese or a free-range egg – every day.

3. Eat three or more servings a day of fresh fruit (a mix of colours).

4. Eat four or more servings a day of whole grains such as rice, rye, oats, wholewheat, corn or quinoa as cereal, breads, pasta or pulses.

5. Eat five servings a day of dark green, leafy and root vegetables such as watercress, carrots, sweet potatoes, broccoli, Brussels sprouts, spinach, green beans or peppers, either raw or lightly cooked.

6. Drink six glasses of pure water, diluted juices or herbal tea each day.

7. Eat oily fish three times a week (anchovies, sardines, mackerel, trout, salmon, herring, kipper and occasionally fresh tuna) – or take a fish oil supplement containing EPA, DPA and DHA if you don't eat fish.

8. Choose whole foods – whole grains, lentils, beans, nuts, seeds, fresh fruit and vegetables, organic if possible.

9. Avoid refined, white and sugary foods and processed foods, particularly those containing artificial additives.

10. Avoid fried, burnt and browned food, hydrogenated fat and excess animal fat.

Get Your Own 100% Health Programme Online

You can go online and get your action plan by visiting *www.patrickholford.com* and completing your online '100% Health Assessment'. The analysis part is free – this assesses your health in similar areas to the questionnaires in Part Two of this book, and gives you a score for each. For a small fee, you can also get a detailed action plan with dietary goals tailored to your needs, along with a personalised supplement plan.

Of course, I'm not suggesting you change your diet overnight to achieve all of these – rather pick one or two each week to implement until you have gradually built up to incorporating them all. The 100% Health Action Plan at the end of this chapter has been designed to help make planning your dietary changes easier.

To help you prioritise which goal to go for first, write your scores for each of the main health areas discussed in Part Two in the box below (or copy the chart on to a sheet of paper). Write beside this which colour zone this correlates to, i.e. red, yellow or green.

Prioritising your dietary goals

If you are in the red zone for any particular area, I suggest you pay particular attention to the dietary goals highlighted in that relevant area. Again, don't overload yourself – just pick one or two each week. If you are in the red for more than one area, prioritise as applicable according to the order they are listed – so blood sugar balance first, then digestion, detoxification, hormone balance, immune function and finally mind, mood and memory. After you've tackled all the reds, next go for the yellows.

To make this easy for you, many of the dietary goals from earlier chapters are repeated here, but there are also some additional goals for you to adopt – these are in italic text.

My Health Scores

	Score (number of yes answers)	Colour Zone (red, yellow, green)
1. Blood Sugar Balance	☐	
2. Digestion	☐	
3. Detoxification	☐	
4. Hormone Balance	☐	
5. Immune Function	☐	
6. Mind, Mood and Memory	☐	

Blood sugar balance

Keeping your blood sugar level balanced is the secret to having abundant energy and staying at your ideal weight.

- Avoid refined, white and sugary foods and processed foods, particularly those containing artificial additives.

- *Choose unrefined low-GL foods and ensure you have some protein with each meal and snack.*

- *Avoid all caffeinated drinks such as coffee, tea and cola. Instead have as many red bush or herb teas as you like.*

- *If you need to lose weight, eat 40 GLs per day until you reach your goal (see Chapter 7 – and also, my book* The Holford Low-GL Diet Made Easy).

Digestion

Problems with digestion, absorption and elimination – as well as food intolerance – can not only create unpleasant symptoms in their own right, they can also undermine your health in other areas.

- Choose whole foods – whole grains, lentils, beans, nuts, seeds, fresh fruit and vegetables, organic if possible.

- Avoid refined, white and sugary foods and processed foods, particularly those containing artificial additives.

- Drink six glasses of pure water, diluted juices or herbal tea.

- *Reduce wheat products in your diet and substitute with oats, brown rice, corn, quinoa, millet and occasionally rye bread.*

- *If you suspect you are intolerant to something you are eating, find out what it is and eliminate it. The most common allergens are wheat and milk, plus gluten grains, eggs, citrus, chocolate and soya.*

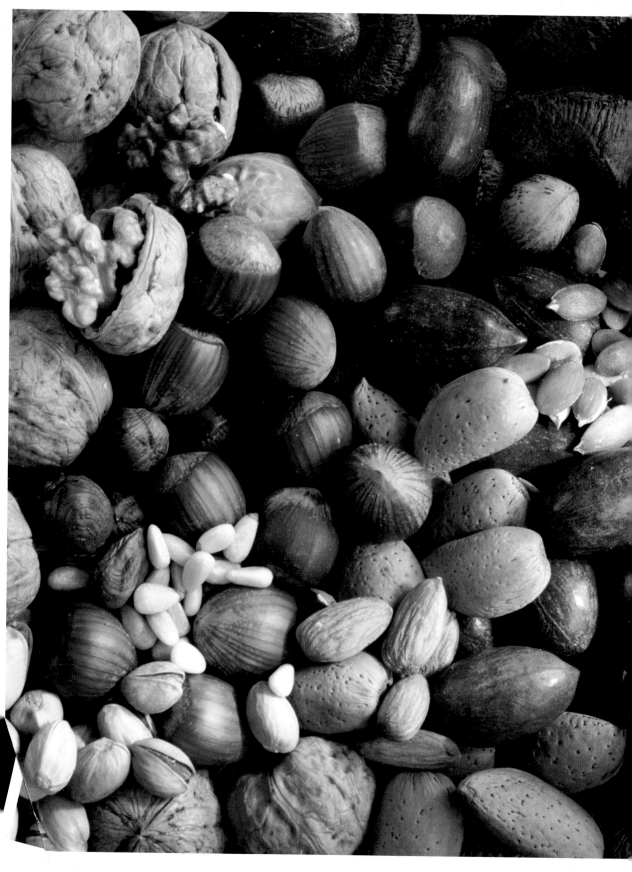

Detoxification

Your ability to detoxify effectively is essential to good health.

- Eat three or more servings a day of fresh fruit (aim for a mix of colours).

- Eat five servings a day of dark green, leafy and root vegetables such as watercress, carrots, sweet potatoes, broccoli, Brussels sprouts, spinach, green beans or peppers, either raw or lightly cooked.

- Avoid fried, burnt and browned food, hydrogenated fat and excess animal fat.

- *Limit your alcohol intake to no more than half a pint of beer or one glass of red wine per day.*

- *Consider following a week's detox programme to give your liver a break and spring clean your body (see page 87).*

Hormone balance

Symptoms of hormonal imbalance can be a thing of the past when your hormones are truly in harmony.

- Eat one handful of fresh seeds or nuts (whole or ground) – or one tablespoon of a cold-pressed seed oil.

- Avoid fried, burnt and browned food, hydrogenated fat and excess animal fat.

- *Aim to have at least half, if not all, of what you eat and drink organic.*

Immune function

Keeping your immune system strong helps to keep you free of illness and allergy.

- Eat three or more servings a day of fresh fruit (aim for a mix of colours).

- Eat five servings a day of dark green, leafy and root vegetables such as watercress, carrots, sweet potatoes, broccoli, Brussels sprouts, spinach, green beans or peppers, either raw or lightly cooked.

- *Limit your alcohol intake to no more than half a pint of beer or one glass of red wine per day. Don't smoke.*

Mind, mood and memory

A sharp mind, happy mood and good memory can be achieved with optimum nutrition.

- Eat one handful of fresh seeds or nuts (whole or ground) – or one tablespoon of a cold-pressed seed oil.

- Eat oily fish three times a week (anchovies, sardines, mackerel, salmon, trout, herring, kipper and occasionally fresh tuna) – or take a fish oil supplement containing EPA and DHA.

- *Have six Omega-3-rich free-range eggs a week.*

Setting a supplement programme

As you'll have read in Part One, while diet can improve your health, you also need supplements to ensure you get optimum levels of all the nutrients you need and reach your goal of 100 per cent health. A basic supplement programme should include:

- A high-strength multivitamin and mineral.
- Extra 1000mg to 2000mg of Vitamin C.
- Omega 3 and Omega 6 essential fats, especially if you don't like oily fish (or don't eat it three times a week) and nuts and seeds each day. Plus...
- An antioxidant formula if you live in a busy city, are or have been exposed to a lot of toxins or are over 50.

Having identified any weak areas in Part Two, you'll also see that there are some additional supplements you can take to help address these. If you have several high priorities, for example you are in the red categories in more than one area, then I suggest you prioritise these in the same order as dietary goals – so balancing blood sugar first, then digestion, detoxification, hormones, immune function and finally mind, mood and memory. See below to recap on the main supplements in each of these areas. These are designed for use while you are bringing this area of your health back into balance – but bear in mind that they are not appropriate for long-term use (i.e. six months plus) without supervision from a nutritional therapist.

To improve blood sugar balance and aid weight loss, consider:
- A basic supplement programme (multi, Vitamin C and essential fats).
- Chromium (200mcg a day) – look for a formula that also contains cinnamon if you are diabetic or have 'insulin resistance', as this enhances the effect of chromium.
- Hydroxycitric acid (750mg a day), plus 5-HTP if weight and/or sugar cravings is your major issue. NOTE: Do not take 5-HTP if you are on anti-depressant medication.

To improve digestion, consider:
- A basic supplement programme (multi, Vitamin C and essential fats).
- A broad-spectrum digestive enzyme with each meal.
- A daily probiotic supplement with both Acidophilus and Bifido bacteria.
- Glutamine (5g a day, dissolved in water, on an empty stomach first or last thing for two weeks).

To aid detoxification, consider:
- A basic supplement programme (multi, Vitamin C and essential fats).
- A daily antioxidant supplement containing at least 1500mcgRE of Vitamin A, 25mg of glutathione (reduced), 200mg of Vitamin E, 10mg of co-enzyme Q10, 10mg of alpha-lipoic acid, 50mg of anthocyanidins, 50mcg of selenium and 10mg of zinc.
- Extra Vitamin C (1–2g a day).
- MSM – which stands for methylsulphonylmethane (1–2g a day).

To reduce inflammation and kill pain naturally, consider:
- A basic supplement programme (multi, Vitamin C and essential fats).
- Extra Omega 3 fish oils (providing 1000mg of EPA a day).

- A daily antioxidant supplement containing at least 1500mcgRE of Vitamin A, 25mg of glutathione (reduced), 200mg of Vitamin E, 10mg of co-enzyme Q10, 10mg of alpha-lipoic acid, 50mg of anthocyanidins, 50mcg of selenium and 10mg of zinc.
- A formula containing combinations of natural anti-inflammatories such as:
  Turmeric, high in curcumin (500–1500mg)
  Boswellia (400–1200mg)
  Ashwagandha (300–1000mg)
  Hop extract, high in iso-oxygene (500–1500mg)
  Olive extract, high in olivenol (60–120mg)
  Ginger (500–2000mg), or eat a 1cm/$\frac{1}{2}$ inch slice of fresh ginger a day
  Glucosamine, for joints (1–3g)
  MSM, high in sulphur (1–3g)

For combination formulas, aim for the lower level in the range. If you are experimenting with individual nutrients or herbs, aim for the higher figure. These are all daily amounts.

To help hormone balance, consider:
- A basic supplement programme (multi, Vitamin C and essential fats).
- To support thyroid, a formula containing tyrosine, iodine, zinc and selenium.
- To relieve a whole range of hormonal symptoms, look for a formula which contains extra Vitamin C, zinc, isoflavones, extra B vitamins and a nutrient called DIM rich in broccoli.
- To aid hormone balance during the menopause, extra Vitamin C (1g a day) in a formula which also contains bioflavonoids.
- For vaginal dryness in the menopause, extra Vitamin E (600mg a day).
- To relieve menopausal symptoms, especially hot flushes, Agnus Castus (20–40mg a day).

To boost immune function, consider:
- A basic supplement programme (multi, Vitamin C and essential fats).
- 2–4g of Vitamin C a day in total and extra while fighting an infection.
- A daily antioxidant supplement containing at least 1500mcgRE of Vitamin A, 25mg of glutathione (reduced), 200mg of Vitamin E, 10mg

of co-enzyme Q10, 10mg of alpha-lipoic acid, 50mg of anthocyanidins, 50mcg of selenium and 10mg of zinc.
- During an infection, consider a daily formula with berry extracts, especially black elderberry extract (at least 100mg) and ginger. Some Vitamin C formulas contain these.
- A daily probiotic supplement.

To improve mood, memory and concentration consider:
- A basic supplement programme (multi, Vitamin C and essential fats).
- To improve memory, supplement extra B vitamins (at least 50mg of B5), TMG (100mg twice a day) with phospholipids phosphatidyl-choline and phosphatidyl-serine and DMAE in a combination formula.
- To boost low mood, supplement 100mg of 5-HTP twice a day. Also take 2000mg of Omega 3 fish oil (providing 1000mg of EPA).
- To boost poor drive and motivation, supplement 500mg of tyrosine twice a day, ideally in a formula containing adaptogenic herbs such as Asian, American and Siberian ginseng, and reishi mushroom extract and B vitamins.

There are also suggestions for other supplements in Part Three – for example to tackle specific health issues such as high blood pressure or high cholesterol, or improve your skin condition. See the Supplement Directory at the back of this book for more on recommended brands and products.

When you have decided on what you want to take – and have found the supplement you want to use (see Supplement Directory for suggestions), write down your supplement programme on your 100% Health Action Plan. If you are confused about what supplements are best for you, my online 100% Health programme will work this out for you (see *www.patrickholford.com*).

Exercise and relaxation

Eating well and ensuring you get all the nutrients you need for optimum health is important. But two other essential parts of the optimum health equation are exercise and relaxation.

Exercise is best incorporated into your everyday schedule – that way you are more likely to stick to it. So walking the kids to and from school instead of driving, or turning cleaning the house into an aerobics workout

My 100% Health Action Plan

Date:

Week: of 100% Health Plan

General Diet Goals	Already doing	This week's goal	Next week's goal
1. Eat one handful of fresh seeds or nuts – or one tablespoon of a cold-pressed seed oil.	☐	☐	☐
2. Eat two servings of vegetable protein – or one small serving of lean meat, fish, cheese or a free-range egg – every day.	☐	☐	☐
3. Eat three or more servings a day of fresh fruit.	☐	☐	☐
4. Eat four or more servings a day of whole grains.	☐	☐	☐
5. Eat five servings a day of dark green, leafy and root vegetables, either raw or lightly cooked.	☐	☐	☐
6. Drink six glasses of pure water, diluted juices or herbal tea.	☐	☐	☐
7. Eat oily fish three times a week or take a fish oil supplement.	☐	☐	☐
8. Choose whole foods – whole grains, lentils, beans, nuts, seeds, fresh fruit and vegetables.	☐	☐	☐
9. Avoid refined, white and sugary foods and processed foods, particularly those containing artificial additives.	☐	☐	☐
10. Avoid fried, burnt and browned food, hydrogenated fat and excess animal fat.	☐	☐	☐

Additional Diet Goals (these are the goals in italic text on pages 141–4)

....

....

....

....

....

Supplements (note what you will take, and the dose, and when you will take it)   am: pm:

....

....

....

....

...is vital to include regular exercise and relaxation in your weekly plan. To help you stick to your goals, photocopy this chart and on it write down what you will do, when you will do it, for how long and on which days: so, for example, you might want to do yoga ('what'), in the morning ('when'), for 30 minutes ('duration'), on a Wednesday and Saturday ('frequency').

Excercise and Relaxation Plan			
What	When	Duration	Frequency

could be more achievable than, say, regular visits to the gym. Exercising with others is also a good way to stay motivated – whether it be joining a local rambling or jogging group or going to a weekly dance class.

Gentle exercise such as yoga or t'ai chi is an excellent way to de-stress while toning and strengthening your body. Most areas hold local classes. There's also another excellent exercise system which you can learn in an afternoon then do on your own at home each day, called Psychocalisthenics. It means strength (*sthenia*) and beauty (*calos*) through the breathe (*psyche*). It only takes 16 minutes a day. I do it myself and find it extremely energising as well as a great way to keep my body toned and fit. See the Resources section for details on the DVD, book and CD, and the workshops we run to teach it.

It is important to include some regular exercise or relaxation in your weekly plan so ensure you take a copy of the chart above and set achievable goals for yourself.

Setting your 100% Health Action Plan

By now, I hope you have a good idea of what you want to do – and the order you're going to do it in. So the time has come to transfer your aims to your 100% Health Action Plan. You can photocopy the chart opposite and above and stick it on your fridge as a reminder of what you are working towards – and also what you have already achieved. I suggest you review it each week and add new goals as you master the existing ones.

Increasing motivation

Making changes is difficult. But achieving optimum health is well worth the effort (just revisit the boxes you ticked at the start of this book to remind yourself of the possible rewards). To help you increase your chances of success, I suggest you:

• Photocopy your weekly plans and stick them to the fridge or kitchen pin board – that way you'll have a regular reminder of your health goals.

• Clear out your cupboards to get rid of any temptations you want to avoid. Also, shop for alternatives so you have, for example, herbal tea or Caro instead of regular tea or coffee, or oatcakes and hummus to snack on instead of biscuits.

• Tell your friends and family and ask for their support.

• Better still, enlist your family and friends to work towards better health with you – if you have someone to share with, you are much more likely to stick to your goals and make progress.

Need extra help?

You can do a great deal to significantly improve your own health by following the advice in this book – optimising your diet, increasing your intake of vital nutrients via supplements and doing regular exercise and relaxation. However, some people may need extra help to address more long-term or complex health problems. If this applies to you, I'd like to suggest some options:

• First, at the end of each chapter or topic I've given recommendations for books which go into much more detail on a range of specific health areas. This may be a good place for you to start finding out more.

• Secondly, I've talked about a few investigative tests which may help you find some answers – for example to identify food intolerances or measure your level of a key health marker called homocysteine. You can order these tests and take the required sample (usually a pin-prick of blood) yourself, which you then send back to the lab for analysis. See the Resources section for more details.

- If you'd like a more detailed plan – along with specific supplement recommendations – then I suggest you visit *www.patrickholford.com* and do a full online health assessment.

- Lastly, you may benefit from some more detailed tailor-made input from a qualified Nutritional Therapist. They will take a full case-history and may well perform additional tests to uncover information about your individual biochemistry and nutritional status. You will therefore receive a diet and supplement programme that's professionally devised to meet your individual needs – plus ongoing support to help you achieve optimum health. Again, you'll find details of how to locate someone in your area in the Resources section at the back of this book.

Keep track of your progress

To keep yourself on track to better health, it's worth reassessing your status in each of the six key areas that we've explored in Part Two. I recommend you do this every two or three months – that way you can see how you are progressing. You can either do this by rubbing out your scores (if you've written them in pencil) and redoing the questionnaires in each chapter (although it's worth keeping a note of your original scores so you have something to compare your new ones against). Or you can go online to my website at *www.patrickholford.com* and click on 'free online health assessment'. You can then fill in the same questionnaires electronically and keep a record of your results.

Join 100% Health

By becoming a 100% Health member my team and I will help you become and stay healthy, keeping you informed, inviting you to seminars and workshops, and helping you find your perfect optimum nutrition programme. See *www.patrickholford.com*.

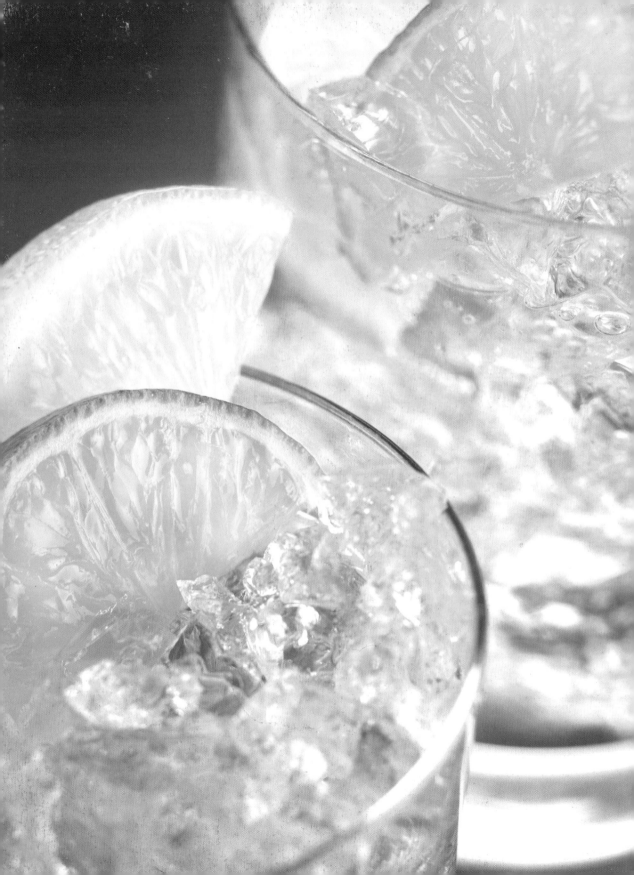

Part Five

Useful Information

Nutrient Fact Files

A guide to what each vitamin, mineral and essential fat does, the most common deficiency signs and the best food sources for each.

Vitamins

Vitamin A (Retinol and Betacarotene)

WHAT IT DOES: Needed for healthy skin, inside and out, protecting against infections. Antioxidant and immune system booster. Protects against many forms of cancer. Essential for night vision.

DEFICIENCY SIGNS: Mouth ulcers, poor night vision, acne, frequent colds or infections, dry flaky skin, dandruff, thrush or cystitis, diarrhoea.

BEST FOOD SOURCES: Liver, carrots, watercress, cabbage, squash, sweet potatoes, melon, pumpkin, mangoes, tomatoes, broccoli, apricots, papayas.

OPTIMUM DAILY AMOUNT: 2500mcg (1500mcg from a good diet; 1000mcg from a supplement).

B1 (Thiamine)

WHAT IT DOES: Essential for energy production, brain function and digestion. Helps the body make use of protein.

DEFICIENCY SIGNS: Tender muscles, eye pains, irritability, poor concentration, prickly legs, poor memory, stomach pains, constipation, tingling hands, rapid heartbeat.

BEST FOOD SOURCES: Watercress, squash, courgette, lamb, asparagus, mushrooms, peas, lettuce, peppers, cauliflower, cabbage, tomatoes, Brussels sprouts, beans.

OPTIMUM DAILY AMOUNT: 35mg (5mg from a good diet; 30mg from a supplement).

B2 (Riboflavin)

WHAT IT DOES: Helps turn fats, sugars and protein into energy. Needed to repair and maintain healthy skin, inside and out. Helps to regulate body acidity. Important for hair, nails and eyes.

DEFICIENCY SIGNS: Burning or gritty eyes, sensitivity to bright lights, sore tongue, cataracts, dull or oily hair, eczema or dermatitis, split nails, cracked lips.

BEST FOOD SOURCES: Mushrooms, watercress, cabbage, asparagus, broccoli, pumpkin, beansprouts, mackerel, milk, bamboo shoots, tomatoes, wheatgerm.

OPTIMUM DAILY AMOUNT: 35mg (5mg from a good diet; 30mg from a supplement).

B3 (Niacin)

WHAT IT DOES: Essential for energy production, brain function and the skin. Helps balance blood sugar and lower cholesterol levels. Also involved in inflammation and digestion.

DEFICIENCY SIGNS: Lack of energy, diarrhoea, insomnia, headaches or migraines, poor memory, anxiety or tension, depression, irritability, bleeding or tender gums, acne, eczema/dermatitis.

BEST FOOD SOURCES: Mushrooms, tuna, chicken, salmon, asparagus, cabbage, lamb, mackerel, turkey, tomatoes, courgettes, squash, cauliflower, whole wheat.

OPTIMUM DAILY AMOUNT: 100mg (50mg from a good diet; 50mg from a supplement).

B5 (Pantothenic acid)

WHAT IT DOES: Involved in energy production, controls fat metabolism. Essential for brain and nerves. Helps make anti-stress hormones. Maintains healthy skin and hair.

DEFICIENCY SIGNS: Muscle tremors or cramps, apathy, poor concentration, burning feet or tender heels, nausea or vomiting, lack of energy, exhaustion after light exercise, anxiety or tension, teeth grinding.

BEST FOOD SOURCES: Mushrooms, watercress, broccoli, alfalfa sprouts, peas, lentils, tomatoes, cabbage, celery, strawberries, eggs, squash, avocados, whole wheat.

OPTIMUM DAILY AMOUNT: 100mg (20mg from a good diet; 80mg from a supplement).

B6 (Pyridoxine)

WHAT IT DOES: Essential for protein digestion and utilisation, brain function and hormone production. Helps balance sex hormones, hence use in PMS and the menopause. Natural anti-depressant and diuretic. Helps control allergic reactions.

DEFICIENCY SIGNS: Infrequent dream recall, water retention, tingling hands, depression or nervousness, irritability, muscle tremors or cramps, lack of energy, flaky skin.

BEST FOOD SOURCES: Watercress, cauliflower, cabbage, peppers, bananas, squash, broccoli, asparagus, lentils, red kidney beans, Brussels sprouts, onions, seeds and nuts.

OPTIMUM DAILY AMOUNT: 25mg (5mg from a good diet; 20mg from a supplement).

B12 (Cyanocobalamin)

WHAT IT DOES: Needed for making use of protein. Helps the blood carry oxygen, hence essential for energy. Needed to make new cells. Essential for nerves.

DEFICIENCY SIGNS: Poor hair condition, eczema or dermatitis, mouth over-sensitive to heat or cold, irritability, anxiety or tension, lack of energy, constipation, tender or sore muscles, pale skin.

BEST FOOD SOURCES: Oysters, sardines, tuna, lamb, eggs, shrimp, cottage cheese, milk, turkey, chicken, cheese.

OPTIMUM DAILY AMOUNT: 25mcg (10mcg from a good diet; 15mcg from a supplement).

Folic acid

WHAT IT DOES: Critical during pregnancy for development of a baby's brain and nerves. Also essential for brain and nerve function. Needed for utilising protein and red blood cell formation.

DEFICIENCY SIGNS: Anaemia, eczema, cracked lips, prematurely greying hair, anxiety or tension, poor memory, lack of energy, poor appetite, stomach pains, depression.

BEST FOOD SOURCES: Wheatgerm, spinach, peanuts, sprouts, asparagus, sesame seeds, hazelnuts, broccoli, cashew nuts, cauliflower, walnuts, avocados.

OPTIMUM DAILY AMOUNT: 600mcg (400mcg from a good diet; 200mcg from a supplement).

Biotin

WHAT IT DOES: Particularly important in childhood. Helps your body use essential fats, assisting in promoting healthy skin, hair and nerves.

DEFICIENCY SIGNS: Dry skin, poor hair condition, prematurely greying hair, tender or sore muscles, poor appetite or nausea, eczema or dermatitis.

BEST FOOD SOURCES: Cauliflower, lettuce, peas, tomatoes, oysters, grapefruit, watermelon, sweetcorn, cabbage, almonds, cherries, herrings, milk, eggs.

OPTIMUM DAILY AMOUNT: 150mcg (100mcg from a good diet; 50mcg from a supplement).

Vitamin C (Ascorbic acid)

WHAT IT DOES: Strengthens immune system – fights infections. Makes collagen, keeping bones, skin and joints firm and strong. Antioxidant, detoxifying pollutants and protecting against cancer and heart disease. Helps make anti-stress hormones, and turns food into energy.

DEFICIENCY SIGNS: Frequent colds, lack of energy, frequent infections, bleeding or tender gums, easy bruising, nose bleeds, slow wound healing, red pimples on skin.

BEST FOOD SOURCES: Peppers, watercress, cabbage, broccoli, cauliflower, strawberries, lemons, kiwi fruit, peas, melons, oranges, grapefruit, limes, tomatoes.

OPTIMUM DAILY AMOUNT: 2000mg (200mg from a good diet; 1800mg from a supplement).

Vitamin D (Ergocalciferol, Cholecalciferol)

WHAT IT DOES: Helps maintain strong and healthy bones by retaining calcium.

DEFICIENCY SIGNS: Joint pain or stiffness, backache, tooth decay, muscle cramps, hair loss.

BEST FOOD SOURCES: Herrings, mackerel, salmon, oysters, cottage cheese, eggs.

OPTIMUM DAILY AMOUNT: 30mcg (15mcg from a good diet and daily sunlight exposure, which provides the equivalent of 10mcg; 15mcg from a supplement and 25mcg in the winter).

Vitamin E (D-alpha tocopherol)

WHAT IT DOES: Antioxidant, protecting cells from damage, including against cancer. Helps body use oxygen, preventing blood clots, thrombosis, atherosclerosis. Improves wound healing and fertility. Good for the skin.

DEFICIENCY SIGNS: Lack of sex drive, exhaustion after light exercise, easy bruising, slow wound healing, varicose veins, loss of muscle tone, infertility.

BEST FOOD SOURCES: Unrefined corn oils, sunflower seeds, peanuts, sesame seeds, beans, peas, wheatgerm, tuna, sardines, salmon, sweet potatoes.

OPTIMUM DAILY AMOUNT: 250mg (50mg from a good diet; 200mg from a supplement).

K (Phylloquinone)

WHAT IT DOES: Controls blood clotting.

BEST FOOD SOURCES: Cauliflower, Brussels sprouts, lettuce, cabbage, beans, broccoli, peas, watercress, asparagus, potatoes, corn oil, tomatoes, milk.

OPTIMUM DAILY AMOUNT: None established. Sufficient amounts made by beneficial bacteria in the gut. No need to supplement.

Minerals

Calcium

WHAT IT DOES: Promotes a healthy heart, clots blood, promotes healthy nerves, contracts muscles, improves skin, bone and teeth health, relieves aching muscles and bones, maintains the correct acid–alkaline balance, reduces menstrual cramps and tremors.

DEFICIENCY SIGNS: Muscle cramps or tremors, insomnia or nervousness, joint pain or arthritis, tooth decay, high blood pressure.

BEST FOOD SOURCES: Cheese, almonds, brewer's yeast, parsley, corn tortillas, globe artichokes, prunes, pumpkin seeds, cooked dried beans, cabbage, winter wheat.

OPTIMUM DAILY AMOUNT: 1000mg (800mg from a good diet; 200mg from a supplement).

Chromium

WHAT IT DOES: Helps balance blood sugar, normalise hunger and reduce cravings, improves lifespan, helps protect cells, essential for heart function.

DEFICIENCY SIGNS: Excessive or cold sweats, dizziness or irritability after six hours without food, need for frequent meals, cold hands, need for excessive sleep or drowsiness during the day, excessive thirst, addicted to sweet foods.

BEST FOOD SOURCES: Brewer's yeast, wholemeal bread, rye bread, oysters, potatoes, wheatgerm, green peppers, eggs, chicken, apples, butter, parsnips, cornmeal, lamb, cheese.

OPTIMUM DAILY AMOUNT: 100mcg (70mcg from a good diet; 30mcg from a supplement).

Iron

WHAT IT DOES: As a component of red blood cells, iron transports oxygen and carbon dioxide to and from cells. Also vital for energy production.

DEFICIENCY SIGNS: Anaemia – e.g. pale skin, sore tongue, fatigue, listlessness, loss of appetite, nausea, sensitivity to cold.

BEST FOOD SOURCES: Pumpkin seeds, parsley, almonds, prunes, cashew nuts, raisins, Brazil nuts, walnuts, dates, pork, cooked dried beans, sesame seeds, pecan nuts.

OPTIMUM DAILY AMOUNT: 20mg (15mg from a good diet; 5mg from a supplement).

Magnesium

WHAT IT DOES: Strengthens bones and teeth, promotes healthy muscles by helping them to relax, so useful for PMS, important for heart muscles and nervous system. Essential for energy production.

DEFICIENCY SIGNS: Muscle tremors or spasms, muscle weakness, insomnia or nervousness, high blood pressure, irregular heartbeat, constipation, fits or convulsions, hyperactivity, depression, confusion, lack of appetite, calcium deposited in soft tissue – e.g. kidney stones.

BEST FOOD SOURCES: Wheatgerm, almonds, cashew nuts, brewer's yeast, buckwheat flour, Brazil nuts, peanuts, pecan nuts, cooked beans, garlic, raisins, green peas, potato skin, crab.

OPTIMUM DAILY AMOUNT: 500mg (350mg from a good diet; 150mg from a supplement).

Manganese

WHAT IT DOES: Helps to form healthy bones, cartilage, tissues and nerves, stabilises blood sugar, promotes healthy cells, essential for reproduction and red blood cell synthesis, required for brain function.

DEFICIENCY SIGNS: Muscle twitches, childhood growing pains, dizziness or poor sense of balance, fits, convulsions, sore knees, joint pain.

BEST FOOD SOURCES: Watercress, pineapple, okra, endive, blackberries, raspberries, lettuce, grapes, lima beans, strawberries, oats, beetroot, celery.

OPTIMUM DAILY AMOUNT: 10mcg (6mcg from a good diet; 4mcg from a supplement).

Molybdenum

WHAT IT DOES: Helps rid the body of the protein breakdown products, strengthens teeth and may help reduce the risk of tooth decay, detoxifies the body from free radicals, petrochemicals and sulphites.

DEFICIENCY SIGNS: Deficiency signs are not known unless excess copper or sulphate interferes with its utilisation. Animals show signs of breathing difficulties and neurological disorders.

BEST FOOD SOURCES: Tomatoes, wheatgerm, pork, lamb, lentils, beans.

OPTIMUM DAILY AMOUNT: None established. Supplementary range between 10mcg and 1000mcg (1mg) per day.

Potassium

WHAT IT DOES: Enables nutrients to move into and waste products to move out of cells, promotes healthy nerves and muscles, maintains fluid balance in the body, relaxes muscles, helps secretion of insulin for blood sugar control to produce constant energy, involved in metabolism, maintains heart functioning, stimulates gut movements to encourage proper elimination.

DEFICIENCY SIGNS: Rapid irregular heartbeat, muscle weakness, pins and needles, irritability, nausea, vomiting, diarrhoea, swollen abdomen, cellulite, low blood pressure resulting from an imbalance of potassium: sodium ratio, confusion, mental apathy.

BEST FOOD SOURCES: Watercress, endive, cabbage, celery, parsley, courgettes, radishes, cauliflower, mushrooms, pumpkin, molasses.

OPTIMUM DAILY AMOUNT: 2000mg (all supplied by diet – no need to supplement).

Selenium

WHAT IT DOES: Antioxidant properties help to protect against free radicals and carcinogens, reduces inflammation, stimulates immune system to fight infections, promotes a healthy heart, required for male reproductive system, needed for metabolism.

DEFICIENCY SIGNS: Family history of cancer, signs of premature ageing, cataracts, high blood pressure, frequent infections.

BEST FOOD SOURCES: Tuna, oysters, molasses, mushrooms, herrings, cottage cheese, cabbage, beef liver, courgette, cod, chicken.

OPTIMUM DAILY AMOUNT: 100mcg (50mcg from a good diet; 50mcg from a supplement).

Zinc

WHAT IT DOES: Component of over 200 enzymes in the body, essential for growth, important for healing, controls hormones, aids ability to cope with stress effectively, promotes healthy nervous system and brain especially in a growing foetus, aids bones and teeth formation, helps hair to bloom, essential for constant energy.

DEFICIENCY SIGNS: Poor sense of taste or smell, white marks on more than two fingernails, frequent infections, stretch marks, acne or greasy skin, low fertility, pale skin, tendency for depression, loss of appetite.

BEST FOOD SOURCES: Oysters, ginger root, lamb, pecan nuts, dry split peas, haddock, green peas, shrimps, turnips, Brazil nuts, egg yolks, wholewheat grain, rye, oats, peanuts, almonds.

OPTIMUM DAILY AMOUNT: 20mg (10mg from a good diet; 10mg from a supplement).

Essential fats

Omega 3 (EPA, DPA, DHA)

WHAT IT DOES: Promotes a healthy heart; thins the blood; reduces inflammation; improves functioning of the nervous system; promotes neurotransmitter balance and reception; relieves depression, schizophrenia, attention deficit, hyperactivity and autism; improves sleep; improves skin condition; helps balance hormones; reduces insulin resistance.

DEFICIENCY SIGNS: Dry skin, eczema, dry hair or dandruff, excessive thirst, excessive sweating, poor memory or learning difficulties, inflammatory health problems – e.g. arthritis, high blood lipids, depression, PMS or breast pain, water retention.

BEST FOOD SOURCES: Mackerel, swordfish, marlin, tuna, salmon, sardines, flax seeds, sunflower seeds.

OPTIMUM DAILY AMOUNT: 1000mg combined EPA, DPA and DHA (400mg from a good diet; 600mg from a supplement).

Omega 6 (GLA)

WHAT IT DOES: Promotes a healthy heart; thins the blood; reduces inflammation; improves functioning of the nervous system; promotes neurotransmitter balance and reception; relives depression, schizophrenia, attention deficit, hyperactivity and autism; improves skin condition; helps balance hormones; reduces insulin resistance.

DEFICIENCY SIGNS: Dry skin, eczema, dry hair or dandruff, excessive thirst, excessive sweating, PMS or breast pain, water retention.

BEST FOOD SOURCES: Safflower oil, sunflower oil, corn oil, sunflower seeds, pumpkin seeds, walnuts, wheatgerm, sesame seeds.

OPTIMUM DAILY AMOUNT: 100mg (50mg from a good diet; 50mg from a supplement).

Resources

General

Food for the Brain Foundation
This is an educational charity which promotes the link between optimum nutrition and mental health. The Food for the Brain Schools Campaign also gives advice to schools and parents on how to make kids smarter by improving the quality of food in and outside of school. Visit *www.foodforthebrain.org*.

Institute for Optimum Nutrition (ION)
ION runs courses including a home-study course and a three-year, part-time Nutrition Therapy foundation degree. For details on courses, consultations and publications, visit *www.ion.ac.uk* or call +44 (0)20 8614 7800.

Nutrition consultations
For a personal referral by Patrick Holford to a nutritional therapist in your area, visit *www.patrickholford.com* and select 'consultations' for an immediate online referral. This service gives details of therapists both in the UK and internationally. If there is no one available near by you can always do an online assessment – see below.

Nutrition assessment online
You can have your own personal health and nutrition assessment online. Visit *www.patrickholford.com* and go to 'free online assessment' for details.

Psychocalisthenics
Psychocalisthenics develops strength, suppleness and stamina, and generates vital energy. The best way to learn it is to do the Psychocalisthenics Training. See *www.patrickholford.com* (seminars) for details on these or call +44 (0)20 8871 2949. Also available is the book *Master Level Exercise, Psychocalisthenics*, and a Psychocalisthenics CD and DVD. For further information see *www.pcals.com*.

Skin-care products
Environ products were developed by cosmetic surgeon Dr Des Fernandes to prevent skin cancer and address the damaging effects of the environment on our skin.

Formulated with scientifically proven active ingredients including Vitamin A and antioxidant Vitamins C, E and betacarotene, which are used in progressively higher concentrations, Environ will help maintain a normal healthy skin, especially when there are signs of ageing, pigmentation, problem skin and scarring. To purchase Environ products, contact Health Products For Life on +44 (0)20 8874 8038, or go to *www.healthproductsforlife.com*. For international enquiries, see *www.environ.co.za*.

Tests

Food or chemical allergy and intolerance tests

YorkTest Laboratories sell a home test kit for food or chemical allergies that requires a pin-prick blood sample you can take yourself at home and then return to the lab for analysis. For more details, visit *www.yorktest.com* or call freephone 0800 074 6185.

Homocysteine test

YorkTest Laboratories also produce a home test kit to measure homocysteine levels. If your homocysteine is high, full instructions are provided to help you reduce it. Visit *www.yorktest.com* or call freephone 0800 074 6185 for details. Also see *www.thehfactor.com* for details of other labs, supplements and to order *The H Factor* book.

Liver test

Another test from YorkTest Laboratories, LiverCheck tests for enzymes that can indicate the extent of any liver damage. This requires a pin-prick sample of blood, which you can take yourself at home. Results are sent with guidelines on how to improve liver health if a problem is detected. For details visit *www.livercheck.co.uk* or call 0800 130 0588.

Gut health test

Again by YorkTest Laboratories, this test measures levels of beneficial and potentially harmful gut bacteria to help assess your digestive health. You will receive a kit with full instructions to return a stool sample to the lab for analysis. Results are provided in an easy-to-understand format for you and a more comprehensive lab report for your health care provider, and you'll also receive guidelines on how to address any digestive problems identified.

Other tests

A full range of biochemical tests are available – for example, to screen for parasites, digestive disorders or toxicity, check hormone levels and assess nutrient status. These tests can be arranged through your local nutritional therapist (see *www.patrickholford.com* for a referral).

Supplement Directory

Finding your own perfect supplement programme can be confusing, but my website, *www.patrickholford.com* offers useful guidance.

The backbone of a good supplement programme is:

- A high-strength multivitamin
- Additional Vitamin C
- An essential fat supplement containing Omega 3 and Omega 6 oils
And...
- An all-round antioxidant complex later in life (over 50)

Herbal, food and nutritional supplements

In this section I list some of my favourite supplements. Supplier details are given at the end.

Aloe vera
This plant from the cactus family has many healing properties and supports healthy digestion, skin and immunity. As such it is a good all-round tonic. BioCare produce an excellent powdered aloe vera. Take two capsules daily. Alternatively, have a measure of aloe vera juice a day.

Antioxidants
A good all-round antioxidant complex should provide Vitamin A (betacarotene and/or retinol), Vitamins C and E, zinc, selenium, glutathione or cysteine, anthocyanidins from berry extracts, lipoic acid, co-enzyme Q10 and resveratrol. My favourite is BioCare's AGE Antioxidant, followed by Solgar's Advanced Antioxidant Nutrients.

Bone health
Minerals such as calcium, magnesium, boron, zinc and silica plus Vitamin C and D all help support bone health. My two favourite supplements are BioCare's Osteoplex and Solgar's Advanced Calcium Complex.

Brain support and phospholipid supplements

The brain needs essential fats (see below), phospholipids such as phosphatidyl choline and phosphatidyl serine, plus other key nutrients to function optimally. Phosphatidyl serine is available in 100mg capsules from BioCare, Solgar and other companies. Phosphatidyl choline (PC) can be found in lecithin granules. BioCare's Brain Food provides all these.

Calming nutrients and herbs

BioCare's Chill Food Formula provides calming hops, passion flower, glutamine and taurine, plus B vitamins. Valerian also aids sleep. Try Solgar's Standardised Valerian Root Extract.

Colon-cleansing and detox supplements

Various herbs and fibres help to cleanse the digestive tract and are a great support for a detox programme. My favourite is BioCare's ColonGuard and Liver Detox Pack.

Digestive enzymes and support

Any decent digestive enzyme needs to contain enzymes to digest protein (protease), carbohydrate (amylase) and fat (lipase). Some also contain amyloglucosidase (also called glucoamylase), which digests glucosides founds in certain beans and vegetables noted for their flatulent effects. BioCare's DigestPro is excellent, as is Solgar's Vegan Digestive Enzymes. DigestPro also contains probiotics.

If digesting milk is a problem, you may lack the enzyme lactase, which breaks down the sugar in milk. If so you can add lactase drops to milk before you drink it. BioCare produce lactase enzyme drops – add 4–8 per pint (570ml) of milk before drinking.

Essential fats and fish oil supplements

The most important Omega 3 fats are DHA, DPA and EPA, the richest source being cod liver oil. The most important Omega 6 fat is GLA, the richest source being borage (also known as starflower) oil. My favourite supplement is BioCare's Essential Omegas, which provides a highly concentrated mix of EPA, DPA, DHA and GLA. BioCare also produces an Omega 3 fish oil supplement which is good value, as is Seven Seas Extra High Strength Cod Liver Oil. Both these products have consistently proven the purest when tested for PCB residues, which are in almost all fish. Cod liver oil also contains Vitamin A. BioCare's GLA Emulsion and Solgar's One-A-Day GLA are good value if you only want Omega 6 fats.

Get Up & Go!

This tasty breakfast shake that you blend with some milk or juice, plus fruit, provides significant amounts of vitamins and minerals plus protein from a blend of rice, soya and quinoa, fibre from rice and oat bran, plus essential fatty acids from sesame, sunflower and pumpkin seeds. At less than 500 calories and low GL, it adds up to a substantial and sustaining healthy breakfast. Available from BioCare.

Hormone-friendly supplements

There are many herbs, vitamins, minerals and phytonutrients, such as isoflavones, that influence hormonal health. For the thyroid, try BioCare's Thyro Complex. For women with hormonal balance problems – whether still menstruating or in the menopause – try BioCare's Female Balance, which contains a range of supportive nutrients including isoflavones.

Immune support and Vitamin C supplements

Vitamin C is the nutrient most vital for keeping your immune system healthy. Also important are zinc, and bioflavanoids and anthocyanidins found in berries, the best of which are elderberry and bilberry. BioCare's ImmuneC provides Vitamin C, bilberry extract, black elderberry extract and zinc. Grapefruit seed extract is also an important part of a natural immune protection programme and is available from Biocare as Biocidin.

Joint support supplements and balms

Combinations of boswellia, curcumins from turmeric, hop extract, olive extract, glucosamine, MSM, plus Omega 3 fats, all help to keep inflammation in check. For stiff or injured muscles or joints I recommend the herb boswellia, as well as ginger, capsaicin and peppermint. For skin healing, ascorbyl palmitate (Vitamin C) and aloe vera are excellent, as is MSM, a form of sulphur. BioCare's Joint Support contains a combination of these nutrients.

Multivitamin and mineral supplements

Supplementing the right multivitamin is the most important supplement decision you make. Most multivitamins are based on RDA levels of nutrients, which are not the same as optimum nutrition levels. The best multivitamin, based on optimum nutrition levels, is BioCare's Optimum Nutrition Formula. The second best is Solgar's VM2000. Both of these recommend two tablets a day. Optimum Nutrition Formula has better mineral levels, especially for calcium and magnesium. Ideally, both should be taken with an extra 1g of Vitamin C. BioCare also makes an excellent children's multivitamin called Optimum Nutrition For Children.

Probiotics

Probiotics are supplements of beneficial bacteria, the two main strains being Lactobacillus acidophilus and Bifidobacterium bifidus. There is quite some variability in amounts of bacteria (some labels say things like 'a billion viable organisms per capsule') and quality. I consider the following supplements to be high quality and well formulated: BioCare's Bifidoinfantis can be taken from birth to weaning; once weaned, babies and children can take BioCare's Banana or Strawberry Acidophilus powder, plain Bio-Acidophilus capsules or Solgar's ABCDophilus. Adults can take Biocare's Bio-Acidophilus, or try BioCare's DigestPro, which contains probiotics along with digestive enzymes. Remember to store your probiotics in the fridge as heat and light can kill off the bacteria.

Weight-loss support

There are three supplements worth considering to support proper metabolism while you are on a weight-loss diet. These are chromium, HCA (hydroxycitric acid) and 5-HTP. BioCare's GL Support provides these. Biocare's Cinnachrome combines chromium with cinnamon. Solgar also have HCA and chromium supplements.

Supplement suppliers

The following companies produce good-quality supplements that are widely available in the UK.

BioCare Available in most health food shops. Tel: +44 (0)121 433 3727. Website: *www.BioCare.co.uk.*

Seven Seas Specialises in cod liver oil, rich in Omega 3 fats. Available in health food stores and pharmacies, or visit *www.sseas.com.*

Solgar Available in most health food shops. Contact Solgar on +44 (0)1442 890355 for your nearest supplier, or visit *www.solgar.co.uk.*

Health Products for Life offers a wide range of health products from supplements to water filters by mail order. Visit *www.healthproductsforlife.com* or call +44 (0)20 8874 8038.

And in other regions

South Africa Bioharmony produces a wide range of products in South Africa and other African countries. For details of your nearest supplier contact 0860 888 339 or visit *www.bioharmony.co.za.*

Australia Solgar supplements are available in Australia. Contact Solgar on 1800 029 871 (free call) for your nearest supplier. Website: *www.solgar.com.au.* Another good brand is Blackmores.

Singapore BioCare products are available in Singapore. Please contact Essential Living on 6276 1380 for your nearest supplier or visit *www.essliv.com.*

New Zealand BioCare products are available in New Zealand. Contact Aurora Natural Therapies, 12a Battys Road, Springfields, Blenheim 7201. Website: *www.aurora.org.nz.*

Index

Note: Page numbers in **bold** refer to diagrams.

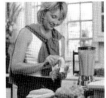 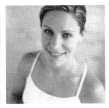 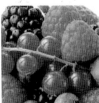
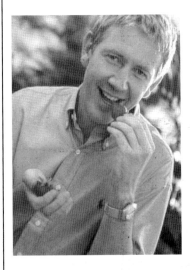